"This book isn't just for women _____ teachers, faculty and administrators who work with _____ and girls It's great for starting honest and transparent conversations about difficult and often embarrassing issues. The statistics are compelling, the ease-of-access to pornography is eye-opening, and the chapter on "your brain on porn" is essential information from which anyone can benefit."

- Becky Tirabassi, Founder of Burning Hearts Inc.
Author and Speaker

"What a powerful book! Working with teen girls and talking candidly with them about the issues they face, I know firsthand many girls are struggling with pornography and the path of destruction it takes them on. It has been difficult for me to find Christian resources that address the issue of pornography and females because it has been stigmatized as a "guy thing." The Christian Woman's Guide to Breaking Free from Pornography gives me the resources I need."

- Katie Wolfe, Founder & CEO of Get Real inC,
www.Getrealinc.org

"This book by far is the best I've seen on the subject of pornography. If you or someone you know is into porn, please tell them about this book. It might be their only hope."

- Scott Mason, Speaker and Author of No Reason to Live
and Beauty & Disgrace, **www.ScottMason.org**

A Christian Woman's Guide to Breaking Free from Pornography

It's Not Just a Guy's Problem

by Shelley Hitz & S'ambrosia Curtis

A Christian Woman's Guide to Breaking Free from Pornography

Body and Soul Publishing

Printed in the United States of America
ISBN-13: 978-0615693897
ISBN-10: 061569389X

Get more resources and connect with the authors here:
www.ChristianWomenandPorn.com

CONTENTS

Introduction

I decided to write this book because I know what it feels like to be caught in the trap of pornography as a Christian woman. Yes, I have struggled with pornography.

It is not something that I am proud of, and to be honest, it is something that I wish never happened, but God is using this dark season from my past for His good.

You see, I travel and speak across the United States to both teens and adults. Once God prompted me to start sharing my testimony of how He freed me from the grips of pornography, teen girls and women began to confide in me their struggles with pornography.

You Are Not Alone If You Struggle with Porn

In fact, pornography is a fast growing problem, even among Christian women. Our goal is to offer hope and resources to help you overcome this trap of the enemy.

Pornography is something that many women are addicted to but not talking about, especially in the church. It is impacting families and marriages and controlling many peoples' lives. For many people, myself included at one time, all they can think about is the next time they will be able to access their computer or the next thrill they will get.

Some get hooked innocently through another person showing it to them or through an ad while surfing the Internet. Others are bored and get drawn into chat rooms or webcams that eventually lead them down the path of getting trapped into a pornography addiction.

Although men are the ones typically drawn to porn due to their visual nature, women are also getting hooked. Even Christian women in good marriages, who are active in ministry, are getting trapped into this sin.

We pray that if you or someone you know is struggling with an addiction to pornography, you will find hope and help within these pages. Ultimately, our hope comes from Jesus Christ, but it also comes from knowing we are not alone and that there is a light at the end of the tunnel. Freedom from pornography is possible!

Now may the God of hope fill you with all joy and peace in believing, that you may abound in hope by the power of the Holy Spirit.

Romans 15:13

~Shelley Hitz

por·nog·ra·phy
noun

obscene writings, drawings, photographs, or the like,
especially those having little or no artistic merit.
(www.dictionary.com)

the depiction of erotic behavior (as in pictures or writing)
intended to cause sexual excitement
(www.merriam-webster.com)

PART ONE: THE REALITY OF PORNOGRAPHY

S'ambrosia Curtis

The night I publicly confessed the secret that I had hidden for over ten years, I must have gone back and forth in my mind dozens of times. I wanted to be free from the sin that so easily entangled me, but I could not stand the thought of my close Christian friends looking down on me. What if my dirty laundry became my "outfit of the day" every time they saw me, or what if they no longer wanted to associate with me once they knew the truth?

Shortly after my confession, when I began to speak one-on-one with others about my struggle with masturbation, I found it difficult to even vocalize the word at all. I would frequently substitute *self-pleasure* for masturbation, because it sounded less repulsive. After all, the connotation of that word is not only negative in the Christian perspective, but it is considered to be straight up dirty, and the fear of being stigmatized and seen as *dirty* was enough to keep me from being completely open about my hidden sin.

The Underlying Issue

Unfortunately, many women find themselves in a similar predicament. They desire to have clean hands and a pure heart before God, which is required to ascend His holy hill, but fear of a tainted reputation causes them to hold onto that which makes them unclean, so they silently slip further into the ever-widening cavern of sexual sin. But how can we be lifted from a pit, if no one knows we are in it? Cloaking our sins may conceal them from the prying eyes of others, but they remain entirely visible to God, and until we learn to view our lives from His perspective, we will not fully comprehend the reality of our spiritual state.

Gaining New Perspective

We all have the propensity to not only lie to others about the state of our hearts, but to lie to ourselves as well. Some of us may refuse to accept the reality of who we have become, because we are afraid of what we will find once we allow the Light to expose our darkest crevices, while others may convince themselves that there are no crevices to be searched. Meanwhile, the sin that we meant to temporarily hide in the closet, ends up taking complete residence in our hearts and turns us into "whitewashed tombs, which look beautiful on the outside, but on the inside are full of dead men's bones and everything unclean" (Matthew 23:27).

Most of us do not realize that this transition has taken place until we discover that communicating with God seems to be more difficult than usual. I counsel quite a few girls regarding sexual addiction, and one commonality I find in every story is that the further they get into their addiction, the less connected they feel to God. 1 John 1:5-9 gives us some perspective on why we feel this way:

> God is light; in him there is no darkness at all. If we claim to have fellowship with him yet walk in the darkness, we lie and do not live by the truth. But if we walk in the light, as He is in the light, we have fellowship with one another, and the blood of Jesus, his Son, purifies us from all sin. If we claim to be without sin, we deceive ourselves and the truth is not in us. If we confess our sins, He is faithful and just and will forgive us our sins and purify us from all unrighteousness.

Facing the Reality of Pornography

At some point in our lives, the fear of losing fellowship with God has got to outweigh the fear of losing face in front of others. Currently, that may seem like an impossible task for you, but reread the last verse in 1 John and be comforted.

If we confess our sins, He is faithful and just and will forgive us our sins and purify us from all unrighteousness.

The One who gave this promise will also be faithful to complete the good work He started in you. Yes, there is a harsh reality concerning the subversive nature of pornography, but the even greater reality is that nothing is too difficult for God.

Chapter 1
Pornography and Women

Part of the challenge we face, when it comes to bringing sexual sin into the light, is the assumption that pornography is a man's problem. Since men are more vocal about their attraction to sexually explicit material, it is easy to see how this misconception has been reinforced. Nevertheless, it is a misconception.

Not Just a Guy's Problem

According to statistics published by Education Database Online in 2011, of the 40 million Americans who regularly visit porn sites, 33% are women. That means that of every three visitors to pornographic websites, one is a woman. Sociologist Michael Kimmel, who studies pornography and teaches sexuality at the State University of New York at Stony Brook says,

> Twenty years ago, my female students would say, 'Ugh, that's disgusting,' when I brought up pornography in class. The men would guiltily say, 'Yeah, I have used it.' Today, men are much more open about saying they use pornography all the time and do not feel any guilt. The women now resemble the old male attitude: they'll sheepishly admit to using it themselves.[1]

How is it that the perception towards pornography among females has changed so significantly? Well, in a 2006 Internet Filter Review study, 70% of women admitted to keeping their cyber activities a secret, and secret activities go hand in hand with hidden sin, one of the enemy's best strategies. The longer we give our sin a dark comfortable environment to grow in, the more uncontrollable it becomes. I would even liken it to the evil alien plant in the musical *Little Shop of Horrors*. The main character Seymour stumbles upon the plant and at first finds it to be harmless, even cute. After a while, he realizes that the plant may not be so cute anymore, as its demands to be fed begins to consume his life. Ultimately, the plant eats not only Seymour, but also his friends. We may believe that we are saving ourselves trouble by hiding what we are doing from others, but in the long run, we are only causing more trouble for ourselves.

The Beginning of a Downward Spiral

To gain a better understanding of pornography's current influence on Christian women, Shelley conducted a survey on her website (www.FindYourTrueBeauty.com) and received responses from 241 Christian girls and women (the full survey can be found in the back of this book). Of the given sample size, 73% of the women had been introduced to pornography. 71% of those who were introduced to pornography had their first encounter with it before the age of 15.

Below, we have provided the various ways these women were first introduced to pornography:

- Internet search – 20%

- Family – 14%
- Friend – 14%
- Magazine – 12%
- TV/movie – 10%
- Ads – 10%
- Boyfriend – 9%
- Internet (accidental) – 6%
- Novels – 3%
- Other – 3%

The progression into pornography usually begins with what seems to be a harmless experience. A friend tells you she found a movie or a magazine under her parents' bed, or maybe you do an Internet search for porn out of curiosity, or you stumble across a sexually explicit scene in a novel you are reading or a movie you are watching. Regardless of which scenario you can claim as your own, the subsequent progression is generally the same for us all.

Dr. Mark R. Laaser, an addictionologist and author of *Healing the Wounds of Sexual Addiction*, suggests that "just looking at porn can never be done without consequences…. Internet porn is the crack cocaine of sexual addiction."[2] All it often takes is just a taste to get the image burned into your memory, and the next thing you know, you find yourself looking for "the hard stuff."

Hard-core vs. Soft-core Pornography

Soft-core pornography is not as graphic or explicit, but it maintains the goal of seeking to arouse the viewer. Generally considered to be the gateway to hard-core pornography, it often leaves more to be desired for the viewer. Examples may include simulated sex scenes, nude photos with strategic cover-ups, or even written descriptions of intimate encounters. Without question, soft-core pornography has infiltrated every aspect of entertainment. Sometimes it can be so blatant that we instinctively feel the need to shield our eyes, but most often it is presented in such a subtle manner that we are completely unaware of the effect it has on us until we realize that our appetite for it has markedly increased. Internet, television, movies, music, magazines, and books have become the primary mediums for soft-core pornography.

The Internet

The largest contributor to the pornography industry, the Internet gives the easiest access to porn, while granting the viewer virtual anonymity. "Studies have shown that women find it easier to click a few buttons on the Internet to search for sexually alluring material. In the absence of a social context, pornography is more appealing to women because there are no social repercussions for using it."[3] Marketers in the pornographic industry are taking advantage of this fact and have boiled their gateway strategy down to a science. Cheryl Wetzstein's *Washington Times* article, "Porn on the web exploding," sheds some light on one particular marketing method.

> If you spend any amount of time on the Internet, it's difficult not to find yourself in the midst of a hard-core porn site – and if you do, you cannot easily leave. A practice called "mouse trapping" means that by clicking out of the site, you'll be hit with a virtually endless series of pop-up ads for other porn sites, and the only way to stop the flood of pornography is to shut the window or turn off the web browser. [4]

This is a genius tactic considering the fact that according to the Sexual Recovery Institute, *sex* and *porn* are among the top

11

five search terms for kids under 18. *Sex* is actually the number one topic for Internet searches, and more than 1.3 million porn sites will pop up at the user's request. [3]

Chat Rooms

Another Internet trap worth mentioning is the chat room. The Internet Filter Review reports that women actually favor chat rooms two times more than men.[5] Mark B. Kastleman, author of *The Drug of the New Millennium: The Science of How Internet Pornography Radically Alters the Brain and Body*, explains that "knowing what we do about the female brain, the chat room is the perfect model to attract women to the Internet." He goes on to share that Internet pornographers have two methods for luring women into chat room relationships:

> [First], the woman starts out with friendly conversation, which eventually leads to romantic talk, then to sexual conversation and hard-core sexual dialogue... the man on the other end will often lead her to the viewing of Internet porn. Exposed to such graphic images right off the bat, most women would reject them, but in the context of a relationship...the woman is slowly coaxed into the world of Internet porn. [Secondly], out of curiosity, a woman may experiment with Internet porn to see what it is all about. This will often lead her to sexually oriented chat rooms, where she will undergo the process of desensitization as described above, and become immersed in the porn viewing/sex addiction cycle. [6]

The Center for Online Addiction also reports that "as men tend to look more for cybersex, women tend to look more for romance in cyberspace. In virtual chat areas... a woman can meet men to form intimate relationships, but like a soap opera, tender moments with a romantic stranger can lead to a passion and progress into sexual dialogue." [7]

Television and Movies

It is almost a given that if you watch any current television show, there will be numerous sexual innuendos floating around. If you happen to miss them in the show, you are almost sure to catch one or two during the commercials. Gary Rose, CEO of The Medical Institute, shared on Focus on the Family (July 8, 2005), that the average teenager spent three to four hours per day watching television, and 83% of the programming most frequently watched by adolescents contained some sexual content. Seven years later, sexual content shows no signs of relinquishing its prominence in television or movies.

Psychological scientists at Dartmouth University recently conducted a study, "Greater Exposure to Sexual Content in Popular Movies Predicts Earlier Sexual Debut and Increased Risk-Taking," to determine the influence of feature films with sexual content on children aged 12-14. Sometimes we tend to believe that sexual content is limited to R-rated films, but after reviewing 684 movies for scenes of activity ranging from passionate kissing to intercourse, they discovered that 68% of G films, 82% of PG, and 85% of PG-13 films contained sexual situations. [8] When combined with the fluctuations of hormones that go hand in hand with puberty, sexual content encourages adolescents to seek sensation.

Personally, movies have always been my weak point. When I was in high school, I would watch R-rated movies and fantasize about casual sex with real and imagined people. By my senior year, my curiosity even led me to sneak out of my parents' house in the middle of the night to meet a boy I met in a chat room. We had been chatting online for a few weeks, when he graciously offered to show me how to make out. I should have known that he was up to no good when he sent me a nude picture of himself and asked me for one, but curiosity got the best of me. With the images of passionate kissing sessions from movies running through my head and the expectation that I would experience something similar, I met this complete stranger in the park. Thankfully, I did not allow things to go as far as he would have liked, but I did do some things that I am ashamed of. The notion of successful casual affairs was cruelly dashed when this particular boy refused to have anything to do with me after that night.

Music

Focus on the Family reported in July 2005 that 42% of the songs on the ten top-selling CDs in 1999 contained sexual content, 41% of which were "very explicit" or "pretty explicit." The analysis of a 2007 study presented in the *Official Journal of the American Academy of Pediatrics* stated that of the content of television shows, movies, magazines, newspapers, and music popular among teens, sexual content was much more prevalent in popular music lyrics than in any other medium. [9]

Think of some of the music you hear on the radio today. Name any song from some of the most popular artists like Lady Gaga, Usher, or Nicki Minaj, and you will find an abundance of sexually explicit lyrics. The problem is not that the lyrics are dirty, but that we are gradually being indoctrinated with messages contrary to the teachings of Christ. The same

14

pediatric study reports that "from music, adolescents gain information about society, social and gender roles, and expected behavior, and they use music to facilitate friendships and social interactions and to help them create a personal identity. It is reasonable to expect, therefore, that the messages conveyed in popular music have significant implications for adolescent socialization behavior." [10]

Worship music is a conduit through which messages can be shared from our heart to God's and vice versa. We sing of our love and devotion to Him, yet we also receive His love as He illustrates His eternal devotion to complete the good work He started within us. Through worship music, I often receive new revelation of the nature of God and His feelings toward me. What messages are we getting from some of the secular songs we listen to? Most songs with sexually explicit lyrics teach women about who they should be and what is expected of them from society. In September 2011, Researchers from Brigham Young University shared that "for girls in particular, [sexually explicit lyrics] can lead them to judge their personal worth on a sexual level only, leading to poor body image, depression, eating disorders, and substance abuse." They go on to conclude that "popular music can teach young men to be sexually aggressive and treat women as objects while often teaching young women that their value to society is to provide sexual pleasure for others." [11] Some studies even go so far as to say that early sexual behavior can be triggered by lyrics of this nature.

Magazines

Ben Shapiro wrote in his book, *Porn Generation: How Social Liberalism is Corrupting our Future*, that the magazines millions of girls subscribe to function as gateway products

15

both for "porn lite" publications like *Cosmopolitan*. When I was in high school, I had a subscription to *Cosmo Girl!* magazine. Upon reading the articles, I began to learn new things about sex and my body, and I became highly fascinated.

As embarrassing as it is to admit, I would even take notes and save them in a box for later. The box has long since been trashed, but I can only imagine how girls, who are not as conservative as I was at that age, would respond. Maybe instead of saving reminders for later, they would impulsively act out their newfound wisdom. This is a hard reality to shrug off, when "most of the teen magazines nowadays revolve around sexual activity," and as Ana Garner of the College of Communications at Marquette University says, "they're training manuals for sex." Regrettably, these are training manuals that three-quarters of adolescent females report reading at least once per month. [12]

Books

Another one of my weaknesses in high school was the mystery novel. Not any mystery novel, but the kind that involved lots of sex, also known as *erotica*. To tell the truth, when choosing a new novel, I would even flip through it first to ensure that it had sexual content before I decided to read it.

In Shelley's survey, 41% of the women said that they read romance novels that contain sexually explicit scenes. Within the 14-18 year old age bracket, over half of the girls (53%) claimed to read these kinds of novels. Some would say that these books are considered female-tailored porn, since they appeal to what women like, whereas most pornography is geared toward men. The key to grabbing a man's attention is to visually stimulate him, but the key to grabbing a women's attention is to stimulate her imagination. Fantasizing goes hand in hand with erotica. With fantasy we do not need to watch hardcore pornography on the screen, because we can easily produce what we want to see in our heads. For this reason, some women would much rather read erotica than watch pornography, but we must be careful not to explain away the pornographic nature of these books. According to the definitions given at the beginning of this book, these types of literature fit the bill for pornography. They are meant to arouse the reader, and that is exactly what they do. Whether you are watching it on the screen or playing it out in your mind's eye, you are engaging in pornography.

Triggering a Response

All of these components of media seem to serve the same purpose: to trigger a response from you. You may have already been aware of some of the influence they had in your life, or you may not have noticed how they affected your life before at all. One thing we are mostly unaware of is how these pornographic images affect our brains and condition us to want more. The next chapter will explain more of what happens in your brain as you are exposed to pornography.

Chapter 2
Pornography and Your Brain

[Pornography] could be more addictive than crack cocaine, because cocaine can be excreted from the body. Pornographic images cannot. They remain, structurally and neurochemically, with a person forever. ~Dr. Judith Reisman (Institute for Media Education)

Unforgettable Images

Being Christian does not automatically spare us from the adverse effects of pornography. If you have ever been exposed to pornography, it is very likely that the images you have seen have been burned into your memory, regardless of how "saved" you were at the time or what your relationship with Christ looks like now. I have only been exposed to hard-core pornography twice in my life, and though what I saw made me physically sick to my stomach, there are certain scenes that I will never be able to erase from my mind. Though I was only in sixth grade at the time of exposure, the images in my mind's eye are just as vivid now as they were then.

Why is it that we can entirely forget certain movies within a few weeks of watching them, yet pornographic images seem to continuously stick around? Normally, when viewing any type of visual stimuli, your brain actively processes what you see in order to make sense of it. Associating what you see with prior knowledge, your brain identifies and categorizes everything that comes before your eyes.

New research has found that "erotic movies can actually quiet the part of the brain that processes visual stimuli."[1] Instead of sending extra blood flow to that region of the brain, explicit movies cause the brain to shunt blood to other regions, such as those responsible for sexual arousal.[2] Gert Holstege, a uroneurologist at the University of Groningen Medical Center in the Netherlands, conducted a study on women to determine their response to material with sex scenes and found that during erotic films, the brain focused on sexual arousal as more important than visual processing.[3]

Because sexual arousal becomes the brain's primary focus, the levels of dopamine in the brain increase. Dopamine, according to *Psychology Today*, is "a neurotransmitter that helps control the brain's reward and pleasure centers. Dopamine also helps regulate movement and emotional responses, and it enables us not only to see rewards, but to take action to move toward them." Elevated levels of dopamine in the brain also produce extremely focused attention, so consequently, "watching pornography causes the viewer to focus intensely on the explicit images at the exclusion of everything else around him."[4]

In the context of intimate relations between married couples, this elevation of dopamine levels generates the same response, causing the couple to be intensely focused on each other during sex.[5] Sex engages not only the physical dimension of a person, but the emotional as well, therefore these sexual experiences are stored in the brain as emotional memories.

Because the brain determines the response of arousal to pornographic images to be the same as a sexual experience, these images are also automatically stored as emotional memories.

If you were to flip through the catalog of your memories, it would be interesting to play the "What Does Not Belong" game. Can you imagine flipping through the line of significant memories, such as the first time you smelled your newborn child or the day you accepted Christ into your life, just before stumbling upon an explicit pornographic image? The thought that something so profane would be categorized with memories so sacred can be a little unsettling. Reviewing our memories from this standpoint, it is easy to determine which ones do not belong, but as far as your brain is concerned, that image indicates that a very intimate experience occurred for you, so it observes no difference between the explicit image and say, your wedding day.

Developing Tolerance and Becoming Desensitized

Dr. Judith Reisman shares:

> Thanks to the latest advances in neuroscience, we now know that pornographic visual images imprint and alter the brain, triggering an instant, involuntary, but lasting biochemical memory trail.... And once new neurochemical pathways are established they are difficult or impossible to delete... these media erotic fantasies become deeply embedded...addicting many of those exposed."[6]

One of dopamine's jobs is to strongly encourage us to engage in experiences that we find rewarding or pleasurable. Dopamine levels increase whenever we engage in stimulating activities. Anything that causes excitement (junk food, jogging, roller coasters, etc.) will cause a spike in dopamine levels. Some situations cause higher spikes of dopamine, but others only give "small hits."[7] Regardless of the intensity of the level of dopamine, with *prolonged* exposure, your brain will begin to adjust and require greater levels of stimulation.[8]

William M. Struthers of Wheaton College compares this process to taking drugs in his book *Wired for Intimacy: How Pornography Hijacks the Male Brain.* "If I take the same dose of a drug over and over and my body begins to tolerate it, I will need to take a higher dose of the drug in order for it to have the same effect that it did with a lower dose the first time." This process is called desensitization, and is the driving force behind tolerance, "which is the need for greater and greater stimulation to experience the same high."[9] Mark Kastleman further explains in his previously mentioned book, that "when one uses pornography to reach climax, the brain desensitizes to the images, habituates to them, and eventually becomes bored. An increase in the variety of images and/or time spent on the Internet is required to maintain stimulation levels."

Taking It to the Extreme

The infamous serial killer Ted Bundy, who murdered over thirty women, granted psychologist James Dobson the opportunity to interview him mere hours before his execution. In the transcript of their conversation, Bundy stressed that

21

though he did not fully blame pornography for the choices he made, he recognized that it helped "mold" and "shape" him into the man he became. He shared:

> Once you become addicted to it, and I look at this as a kind of addiction, you look for more potent, more explicit, more graphic kinds of material. Like an addiction, you keep craving something which is harder and gives you a greater sense of excitement, until you reach the point where the pornography only goes so far – that jumping off point where you begin to think maybe actually doing it will give you that which is just beyond reading about it and looking at it.[10]

Bundy's situation is undoubtedly on the extreme side of the spectrum, and not everyone will respond to pornography the way he did, but it is nevertheless a reality for many. We are all built differently neurochemically, so for some, the addiction truly can reach this extreme.

Remember our friend dopamine? This catalyst behind the addiction process is produced by certain groups of cells in the brain. These cells have receptors called autoreceptors that "help limit dopamine release when the cells are stimulated."[11] Concentration of autoreceptors varies from person to person, but the general rule is that the fewer number of autoreceptors present, the more likely the person will be to seek out new and thrilling experiences. David Zald, an associate professor of psychology states that "the fewer available dopamine autoreceptors an individual has, the less they are able to regulate how much dopamine is released when the cells are engaged. Because of this, novelty and other potentially rewarding experiences, that normally induce dopamine release, will produce greater dopamine release in these individuals."[12] These types of people typically need lots of stimulation in order to reach their dopamine threshold; therefore the entire tolerance process is intensified for these individuals, so they tend to act out in more extreme ways. For most people though, "acting out" is usually demonstrated in either engaging in various sexual relationships or masturbation.

"The Jumping off Point"

59% of the women in Shelley's survey confessed that their involvement with pornography led to other things, such as masturbation or sexual intercourse. Masturbation is defined by Merriam-Webster as "erotic stimulation especially of ones own genital organs... achieved by manual or other bodily contact exclusive of sexual intercourse, by instrumental manipulation, occasionally by sexual fantasies, or by various combinations of these agencies." Adding to the pleasure aspect of the dopamine release, masturbation can be just as addictive as pornography.

My battle with the addiction cycle was not with watching hardcore pornography, but with fantasy and masturbation. There were seasons in my life when it seemed like I had it beat, but if I watched a romantic movie with an explicit sex scene or developed a crush on someone, it would trigger my fantasies, which would in turn trigger the need to masturbate. For the sake of clarification, when I did masturbate, I never penetrated the vaginal area. For a long time I had convinced myself that it was not actually masturbation, but in truth, *any* self-stimulation of the genitals is masturbation.

The Great Masturbation Debate

I first confessed my struggle with masturbation by posting a note on Facebook. It is not recommended that confessions be given to this extreme, but I personally felt led to do it this way. After grappling with this sin for so long, I felt that drastic action was necessary to expose it. Though I received a great response from women who personally messaged me to "come clean" about their struggles, I did get a message from a male who believed that there was nothing wrong with masturbation.

I have had many conversations with men and women alike regarding the issue of masturbation and whether or not it is a sin. Do I believe that children who get curious and "explore" their bodies are sinning? No, but for me, masturbation was always connected to lust and fantasy, and Jesus makes it very clear in the Sermon on the Mount that lust is sin (Matthew 5:28). Each time you fantasize about having sex with someone that you are not married to, in God's eyes, you are committing adultery with them. Physically, I am still a virgin, but I have no right to hold that over anyone's head because as far as God is concerned, I have committed adultery, or fornicated, several times. This standard of living far exceeds the standard that most of us set for ourselves, but if we would learn to live by it, we would discover what true purity looks like. If only we would allow God's Word to illuminate our heart in this manner, to see sin as He does, we would not try so hard to make excuses for pleasuring ourselves.

The Idolatry of Masturbation

While masturbating without experiencing lust is something that I have never practiced, it can be done. Some people masturbate simply because they are bored or it has become a mindless habit, while others feel it releases sexual tension, among various other reasons. We have already established that sex is interpreted by the brain to be just as much of an emotional experience as a physical experience, right? Well, having sex with yourself requires no emotional attachment, so the more you engage in self-pleasure, the more likely you are to become comfortable with having emotionless sex. The detrimental effects of this kind of behavior were realized for one man the hard way:

> As sex becomes little more than another way to meet your own physical needs, the tendency is to ignore the emotional needs of your spouse as well. She becomes nothing more than an object for your sexual satisfaction. In my own marriage, this led to a point where I did not need my wife physically or emotionally, so I started to completely shut down from her. This led to separation and divorce after 13 years of marriage. [13]

The question that remains to be answered is whether or not masturbation, without the lust factor, is sin. As Christians, we know that worship belongs to the Lord alone. Whenever the main object of our affection or satisfaction is not God, we are committing idolatry. An easy test to discover what you truly worship is to hold your heart up to this definition: "We worship whatever rules our time, energy, thoughts, longings, and choices...We want to be mastered by the objects of our worship, and indeed we are."[14] If pleasuring yourself has become something that governs your time, energy, thoughts, longings, and choices, it is an idol, and worshiping idols is the equivalent of committing adultery with God. Recall the story of Hosea, whom God told to marry a prostitute named Gomer. She was unfaithful to her husband and knew many other lovers throughout their marriage. Their relationship was a symbol to all of Israel of how the nation's worship of idols was an act of adultery against God. Likewise, we must be careful not to become like Gomer and forsake our first love for idols.

Put to death, therefore, whatever belongs to your earthly nature: sexual immorality, impurity, lust, evil desires and greed, which is idolatry.

Colossians 3:5

Dealing with Sexual Abuse

In my experience with counseling girls who struggle with masturbation, I have noticed a trend in the number of them that also experienced sexual abuse as a child. I am convinced that this connection is no coincidence. Unfortunately, at the time of sexual abuse, the child's sex drive is awakened. Something that was meant to be opened within the context of a loving, marital relationship was callously forced open too soon, and the child is left wondering how to cope.

The effects of this "awakening" continue to unfold throughout adulthood. Some women I have spoken to will masturbate excessively, while others will engage in sex with various men. In the *Childhood Sexual Abuse* reference handbook, Karen Kinnear explains that "adults who have been sexually abused as children may exhibit sexual acting out or promiscuous behavior. They may be trying to overcome feelings of powerlessness that they experienced as children, or they may be confused over the boundaries of behavior that define affection, sex, and abuse."[15]

It is important to note here, that if you have experienced sexual abuse as a child and currently struggle with sexual behavior, it is not your fault. Do not allow the enemy to make you feel guilty for the sexual urges you felt as a child or that you may feel now. Those urges do not mean that you enjoyed the abuse or that you are a bad person. They are a natural response that many women face. Please rest assured though, that you can still be set free from the cycle. Just like Hosea did to Gomer in Hosea 2:14-16, the Lord will allure you and lead you into the wilderness to speak tenderly to you. He will cleanse you with hyssop and give back what was taken from you, and you will again respond to Him as in the days of your youth.

Doing What You Do Not Want to Do

We all long to encounter God in the way described above, but because we are also aware of our sin, we feel ashamed. This feeling of guilt may even be the reason some of you picked up this book. In Romans 7:15-24, Paul shares a personal inner struggle with which you may be able to identify:

I do not understand what I do. For what I want to do I do not do, but what I hate I do... For I have the desire to do what is good, but I cannot carry it out. For I do not do the good I want to do, but the evil I do not want to do – this I keep on doing. Now if I do what I do not want to do, it is no longer I who do it, but it is sin living in me that does it. So I find this law at work: Although I want to do good, evil is right there with me. For in my inner being I delight in God's law; but I see another law at work in me, waging war against the law of my mind and making me a prisoner of the law of sin at work within me. What a wretched man I am! Who will rescue me from this body that is subject to death?

Paul perfectly sums up the prayer that I found myself repeatedly praying over the course of ten years. *Why do I keep doing what I know I should not do? Why can I not just stop?* This feeling of guilt can lead a person struggling with pornography to make radical decisions toward repentance and freedom, or the shame can lead you right back into the cycle.

It can make you feel so bad that your brain will attempt to keep you from feeling "low," by getting you "high" again, off of pornography. Even though watching pornography ultimately causes you to feel down, you will constantly need to interact with it in order to feel good. This is most likely why 44% of the women who claimed they were addicted to pornography in Shelley's survey also admitted to feeling hopeless in trying to overcome their addiction.

Finding Hope in a Hopeless Situation

Paul ends this section of scripture with the encouraging statement, "Thanks be to God who delivers me through Jesus Christ our Lord!"

Thanks be to God, that the slough of despair's grip is no match for the mighty right hand of the Lord. Thanks be to God, that we have hope because we know He is mighty to save. Did Jesus not say that He came to set the captives free and bind up broken hearts? Thanks be to God for giving us the victory and ensuring that we are never alone.

Chapter 3
Pornography and the Church

Sexual immorality is frequently listed in the Bible as a detriment to ourselves and our relationship with God.

Flee from sexual immorality. All other sins a person commits are outside the body, but whoever sins sexually, sins against their own body.

1 Corinthians 6:18

It is God's will that you should be sanctified: that you should avoid sexual immorality; that each of you should learn to control your own body in a way that is holy and honorable, not in passionate lust like the pagans, who do not know God.

1 Thessalonians 4:3-5

But among you there must not be even a hint of sexual immorality, or of any kind of impurity, or of greed, because these are improper for God's holy people....For of this you can be sure: No immoral, impure or greedy person –such person is an idolater– has any inheritance in the kingdom of Christ and of God.

Ephesians 5:3,5

God makes it very clear to believers that we should have no part in sexual immorality. The scripture listed above, as well as 1 Corinthians 6:9-10, even states that those who choose a sexually immoral lifestyle, among other things, will not inherit the kingdom of God. Suddenly, it makes sense why we are so strongly encouraged to *flee* from sexual immorality (1 Cor. 6:18).

Matters of eternity are at stake.

With God's opinion on sexual immorality being so clearly defined in the Word, one would think that the Church would be a big advocate for ensuring that its members are properly equipped to resist temptation, yet the influence of pornography is just as dominant in the Church as it is in the world, and it is showing no signs of slowing down. Thirty-four percent of churchgoing women say that they *intentionally* visit porn websites online.[1] Even worse, according to a confidential survey of evangelical pastors and church lay-leaders, 64% confirmed that they struggle with sexual addiction or sexual compulsion themselves.[2] Sexual immorality is running rampant through the Body of Christ, leaving traces of filth on a pure white garment.

In a presentation to the Senate Subcommittee on Science, Technology, and Space, Senator Sam Brownback stated:

> Over the last few decades, the nature of, and access to sexually explicit material in the marketplace has been radically transformed and expanded. With the advent of the Internet and video technology, the problem of addiction to sexually explicit material has grown exponentially in size and scope.[3]

It is clear that the voice of the pornographic industry is getting louder, but what we need are the voices of opposition, the voices of the saints. So the question of the hour is, what is the Church going to do about this?

The Spiritual Realm

In the previous chapter I discussed the psychological aspect of dealing with pornography. There is another realm where the pornographic industry has influence, and that is the spiritual realm. Before the Church creates another program to help people overcome addictions, we must realize that the battle we face simply cannot be won on the natural front alone. Our primary line of defense is a spiritual one, and the best way to defeat our spiritual enemy is to know how he works. Two terms that lend themselves well to understanding how the enemy works in the spiritual realm are *foothold* and *stronghold*.

When we are first exposed to temptation and we give in, the enemy gets what is called a foothold. This simply means that he has an access point to your heart that he will continue to use to gain full entry. If we put it in terms of mountain climbing, the enemy is hanging off of a cliff by one hand. At this point, it is very easy to remove him by repenting and casting away whatever sin gave him access, but if repentance does not happen at that point, and the sin is repeated, the enemy gains another foothold. Now he has both arms on that cliff. Because his legs are not involved yet, it is still fairly easy to remove him, but if allowed, he will secure himself on that cliff and begin working on what is called a stronghold.

A stronghold is like a fortress that would be used in war. Once the enemy has gotten a firm foothold, he begins building a stronghold to claim his territory and get anyone who opposes him out. Removing a stronghold requires much more energy than flicking a person off of a mountain. In the same way, the stronghold of pornography that the enemy has set up within the church is going to take a lot of work.

The Weapons of Our Warfare

Thankfully, it is not by *our* might or *our* power that we remove these strongholds, but by the Spirit of the Lord (Zechariah 4:6). We bring Christ our weakness, our inability to break through the enemy's walls, and He gives us His strength. Through His strength we discover that we have divine power to completely demolish strongholds (2 Corinthians 10:4). Jesus told His disciples that whatever they bound on earth would be bound in heaven, and whatever they loosed on earth would be loosed in heaven (Matthew 16:19, 18:18). This is our reality as well, and all of this is done through prayer. Prayer is essential in tearing down the strongholds of the enemy.

As individuals, we have a responsibility to continually lift our concerns to the Father in prayer. We must demonstrate a reliance on Jesus to set us free from the sins that beset us. Prayer is our connection to the Father and grants us access to His authority. Corporately, we need to support one another in prayer (intercession) and pray for the righteousness of God to prevail in the Body of Christ. In the place of prayer, we receive specific strategy not only concerning how to pray, but we also receive strategy for how we need to respond.

A Desire for More Teaching

Forty-four percent of churchgoers stated that they wanted to hear more scriptural teaching from their pastors on the subject of sex, but only 22% of pastors feel they should spend more time on the topic.[4] There could be various reasons for why this is the case, but as a *Christianity Today* analyst said, "Perhaps this desire for more biblical exposition on sexual issues exists because pastors are not speaking forcefully or clearly enough, while exposure to sexual images and messages in today's media is ever more heightened."[5]

Iron Sharpening Iron

One of the primary aims of the Body of Christ gathering together is to sharpen one another and spur each other on to love God and others more, so it is not only the pastor's job to communicate the truth about this issue. According to James 5:16, we are to confess our sins to each other and pray for each other when we gather together. We were never meant to go through this battle on our own.

In the subsequent sections, following the personal testimonies of young women and women like yourself, Shelley will give some strategies on how we can find deliverance as individuals as well as a Body.

PART TWO:
TRUE STORIES OF STRUGGLE AND FREEDOM

Whenever we encounter problems in life, it is important for us to remember that we do not overcome for the sake of our own freedom, but to help others receive the same freedom. On the following pages you will find testimonies of women who have overcome their struggle with pornography or masturbation. Each and every one acknowledges that this process is one of *daily* choosing to die to self. We pray you find encouragement to do the same as you read their stories.

Chapter 4
Set Free to Set Others Free

S'ambrosia

By the time I reached junior high, my thought life was out of control. Being boy-crazy at that age was a given, but when coupled with my overactive imagination and the influence of popular media, my thoughts would go to places I would never have dared to go in reality.

Struggling to Keep Up Appearances

As time progressed, merely thinking about sex wasn't enough. Desiring to get more stimulation from the fantasies, I began to masturbate. I knew it was wrong, but because it had become a habitual practice for me, it seemed impossible to stop...no matter how many times I promised God that I would. For over 10 years I struggled with this and never told anyone. I didn't know of any girls that struggled with the issue, and I was ashamed of what they would think of me if I told them that I did. This wasn't the kind of thing good little Christian girls did, and as an extremely sheltered pastor's kid, I had a reputation to maintain.

The Breaking Point

One night in college, after falling into temptation yet again, I got so frustrated with my perpetual status as a slave to my flesh that I decided to kill this sin once and for all. I personally believe that when you deal with sin, you have to take drastic measures, since sin doesn't hold anything back when it has you in its clutches. Matthew 18:8 even says to cut your hand off and throw it away, if it causes you to sin! That's pretty drastic.

Of course I didn't cut my hand off (and neither should you), but I knew that I needed to have that same type of mentality when approaching my sin, so after repenting to the Lord for the last time, I got on Facebook and confessed my hidden sin in a note. I knew that once I confessed, I'd be able to step out of the darkness, and I wanted to expose the sin myself instead of waiting for it to expose me. Do you know what sin does when it's exposed to the light of God? It flees. That's why the enemy tries so hard to keep us from confessing our sins. He knows that as soon as the light of Christ touches the dark places of our hearts, they can no longer stay.

Setting Captives Free

Do you know what happens when members of the Body confess their sins to one another? They open the door for others who struggle with the same problem to open up as well. Upon reading my note, people started coming out of the darkness themselves and confessed to me that they had been struggling with the same thing. All that time we could have been walking together in the light, but because of fear, we struggled alone in silence. Not cool.

I wrote that note in August of 2008, and I'm still completely free! God has taken what was a season of bondage for me, and turned it into a ministry that allows me to share my testimony and help others overcome.

Overcoming Temptation

I won't say that the temptation hasn't come for me to revert back to my old habits, because it most definitely has, but the Lord has so graciously strengthened me through His Spirit to be able to resist those temptations. He alone is my primary source of freedom, but I also have a responsibility to guard my heart by watching the types of things I feed my flesh, and I take that seriously.

For instance, I will not allow myself to watch movies with ANY sexual content, because I know it will trigger temptation. It is now a force of habit for me to automatically check the back of the movie case for ratings. If sexual content is listed, I put it down and keep on walking. Because society looks at sex differently than we should, there may not be a sexual rating even though sexual content is in the movie, so you have to be careful. Sometimes I make errors in judgment and come across scenes that I shouldn't watch, and though I would like to say I always immediately turn it off, I do find myself making excuses for why I think I can handle it. The problem with that is that when I do allow myself to compromise, it always seems to begin a trend of compromises. There have been a few times that I've started with a small compromise and then within the week, I found myself watching rated R films again. Beware of compromise.

Battlefield of the Mind

In those moments of weakness, when I allow the enemy to advance into the territory of my mind through media, I have a second line of defense. The movies themselves don't make me want to masturbate; the stories I play out in my imagination do, so what I have to do is take captive my imagination (1 Cor. 10:5). As soon as the thoughts begin to turn towards inappropriate sexual behavior, I take them captive. This is key. You must not allow it to get even a foothold in your mind. Take it captive and replace it with something that fits the requirements given in Philippians 4:8:

Whatever is true, whatever is noble, whatever is right, whatever is pure, whatever is lovely, whatever is admirable – if anything is excellent or praiseworthy – think about such things.

When you first begin practicing this, it will be difficult, but because I've made it a habit, it truly comes naturally to me now. If you allow the Holy Spirit to keep perfecting His work in you, you will find that the battle isn't as hard as it once seemed. His strength is made perfect in your weakness, so one day you'll look at how far you've come from where you were, and you'll know that it's all because of Him.

Chapter 5
On a Journey with God

Angie

I grew up in a Christian family, and "knew" God since I was really little. I spent most of my childhood going to different churches and Bible studies, so I knew all the words to say and I knew how to perform. I was the "perfect little lady" for everyone, or at least that's what I wanted to show.

Becoming a Slave

At twelve I discovered something that later became my addiction, my drug, and my god. Masturbation. At first it looked like I was in control, but years later it became something I couldn't control at all. Like a drug, my body would ask me for my daily shot, and if didn't do it, I would have withdrawal symptoms such as bitterness, a little hand shaking, depression, anxiety, etc. It got to a point when I couldn't spend one day without my shot of masturbation. I would lie in my bed in the middle of the night crying out to God because I was doing something that my spirit didn't want, but my body begged me desperately. I was a slave to masturbation.

By seventeen I was a total mess even though it looked like I had everything together. In reality I didn't know how to connect with others, I frequently thought about ending my life, I was depressed all the time, and I didn't want to have intimacy with others because I only knew how to be "intimate" with myself. I felt so ashamed that I couldn't even talk to God anymore. I had also started watching porn. It got to a point when I didn't even feel shame or pain anymore.

The Gradual Process of Change

I wish this could be the part of the story with the happy ending, where I say that one day God came into my life and took it all, or that I never masturbated or watched a porn video again. No, for me it has been a daily, hurtful process of accepting that masturbation and porn are *not* going to fill the deep void in my heart and the *only* one that is able to fill it is God; of confessing and repenting; of facing my deepest emotions and pain (some that I didn't even know were there) and slowly letting God take care of that; of being honest with God, myself, and others; of going to counseling; and of accepting that giving in to masturbation and porn is idolatry (because you run to it instead of running to God).

I no longer struggle with porn, but I do struggle with masturbation some days. I know that God has the power to take all of this away, He has already overcome it all at the cross, but I also believe that He is a gentleman, and He does not do anything without our permission. He wants us to collaborate with Him. We need to feel the pain of growing and changing, the pain of metamorphosis, the pain the caterpillar feels while becoming a beautiful butterfly. If we don't experience it, life wouldn't make sense at all.

God loves you even if you fall. There is nothing you can do or not do that is going to make Him love you less. We are the ones hurting ourselves by the decisions we make, by running away from Him and His love. I remember the answer from God every single time I asked him things like, "Why am I in this situation?"

His answer was, "I love you."

41

"Why can't I feel You?"

"I'm here, have always been, and will always be. I love you."

I would say to God, "I hate You."

He would say, "I love you, my beautiful princess."

"You are not listening to me."

"I listen to every word that comes from your mouth."

"Didn't You see what I just did?"

"Yes, I did see, and I love you anyway."

"I feel far from You."

"Nothing can ever separate you from my love, because I love you with an everlasting love."

Blessed Assurance

The only thing I'm sure of in this life is that God loves you, and He loves me. Let him draw you closer to His heart. If you are struggling with porn, masturbation, or any sexual addiction, let me tell you that I know how you feel because I have been there, and I'm still a work in progress. Remember, we need to collaborate with God if we want to overcome this struggle. God is the only one that can turn our pain into something really wonderful.

Chapter 6
Turning My Weakness into Strength

Sarah

Although I wasn't a believer as a young, married adult, I hated pornography. Regardless, my husband liked to look at pornography and wanted me to watch, so I did.

Lasting Impact

I struggled with getting the images out of my mind, but at the same time I was drawn to them. As a result, I felt shame and guilt, but I also felt too embarrassed to confide in anyone. When I became a believer, the images would still hit me out of the blue, so I knew that it was more than just a struggle in my mind. I was actually fighting a spirit of immorality. I began to realize that in order to overcome this spirit, I actually had to do battle.

Submitting Myself to God

Daily, I would lift the members of my body to God and His righteousness.

And do not go on presenting the members of your body to sin as instruments of unrighteousness; but present yourselves to God as those alive from the dead and your members as instruments of righteousness to God.

Romans 6:13 (NASB)

We are destroying speculations and every lofty thing raised up against the knowledge of God, and we are taking every thought captive to the obedience of Christ.

2 Corinthians 10:5 (NASB)

I cried out to God for deliverance, and He helped me. Every time an image would enter my mind, I would sing, quote scripture, bind my mind to Christ, and put on His armor to protect me from all the fiery darts the enemy would throw my way. I didn't win the battle every time, but I kept getting back up until I had the victory. Because of this struggle, I became stronger and stronger and I learned to battle against the enemy.

Hearing from the Lord

One day the Lord spoke to me when I was crying out, and He told me that my weakness would be my strength. The enemy always tries to plant negative seeds in the area the Lord wants to use for His Kingdom. The Word says that in our weakness His strength is manifest; I found this to be very true. Whenever my mind would flash back to those negative images, I would picture Jesus and beautiful things. As a result, I not only grew closer to Jesus, but I developed a very strong seer gift which I use to help others both in the Kingdom and in evangelism.

Although shame is probably what kept me bound the longest, I was really set free knowing that God would use my weakness as my strength. I didn't need to wallow in guilt anymore, because I could release my guilt to Jesus, and His bountiful and never-ending grace was always there.

Chapter 7
A Testimony in Progress

Hannah

I developed sexual thoughts and began to masturbate when I was about eleven. Unaware of the damage it was doing to me, I continued thinking that this was what pleasure was supposed to feel like, so I would do it to relieve myself of pain, stress, frustration, and anger. It was my "good escape," and I became addicted to the feeling.

Good Feelings Turn to Guilt

This was until I realized I was becoming more embarrassed by it and feeling guilty about it for some reason. I finally found out that it was a sexual sin, so I asked God –no, I begged God– to help me get out of that rut. I even thought of not marrying, for fear this sin would become a generational sin. The embarrassment was indescribable. It was as if I was putting my Christian family to shame. I didn't know who to turn to for help.

I knew I wanted to serve God and I wanted to be a blessing to others, but I didn't know how to do it without being completely free myself. I had heard stories that some people with my problem had to go through deliverance to cast out the evil spirit that was binding them. I had also heard of the importance of telling someone, so they can keep you accountable, but both solutions meant *exposure,* and I wasn't quite ready to let people in on my secret yet.

Looking for a Confidant

At first I thought of handling it on my own because I battled with the fear of being judged. Where I come from, people don't talk about masturbation or porn. It's a problem in our society, but we generally don't talk about it. I grew up in an environment where sex wasn't discussed in church until you were well into adulthood, so I was looking for that one I could confide in, who was not only spiritual, but also non-judgmental because she had gone through the same pain, shame, and low self esteem. As I gathered courage and began to understand the importance of transparency, I began telling people (albeit people far away via the Internet) and told myself to trust God to heal the inner wounds I had caused.

God Demonstrates His Faithfulness

God has been so good. He sent someone to talk to me about my experiences, and now He's given me the opportunity to share my story with you. He has never once left me alone in my struggles, and He's given me this incredible patience to stop and continually offer my life and body to Him. There are times when my thoughts still wander, but God knows I'm trying.

I wouldn't say that I'm completely free right now, and there are high and low points in my journey, but God is continuing to gently nudge me to give up my old lifestyle of watching too much TV, so I can spend more time in His presence. This is a testimony in progress, but the feeling you get when you start to trust God is amazing.

I was once lost, but now am found.

Chapter 8
A Struggle for Purity

Dana

I hate that I've seen porn. It did nothing to better my life, nothing but add struggle to my already struggle-ridden life. I accepted Christ in my early twenties, so I'd already been exposed to porn and masturbation, and did not know until long after my conversion how toxic they were. Even though I never acquired an addiction to porn, it still did its damage. Something I realized fully when I got married.

Keeping the Marriage Bed Pure

My husband and I made the commitment that our relationship would be porn and masturbation free. And for the most part, it is. We don't actively seek out these things, but I still live with the guilt—mostly because porn from my past frequently pops into my mind while we are being intimate. This is not how I want my marriage bed to be made, but I admit that more often than not I am too weak in those moments to take those thoughts captive. What I have to do is pray before every bedroom session so that I am completely there and not haunted by ghosts of porn past. Still, I don't do this as often as I should, which is not doing my love life any favors.

Keeping My Mind Pure

Another struggle for me is the porn I create for myself. During my single years I daydreamed endlessly about falling in love and, of course, doing it (again, thanks to my exposure to porn I had lots of ideas floating around up there). I did this so often that it became the most comforting way for me to drift off to sleep. Fast forward to married life and my go-to imaginary world is now flagrant adultery. I struggle because I must take all thoughts captive, even at the end of the day when I am tired, and all I want to do is dream up an imaginary stud. My struggle to keep mentally pure still irks me, but the harder I work at it, the easier it becomes.

Holding on to God's Promises

My true wish is that I only have desire for my husband, the promise God has for all of us who put Him first in our marriage. I wholeheartedly believe this promise, but being exposed to porn has made this hard to attain. This is one of many struggles in my walk with Christ, but I know if I let go, He will help me just enough for me to conquer this sin. I think it is important to remember that God is there to give you the strength, but it is ultimately up to you to decide to overcome.

Chapter 9
Breaking Free from Sexual Sin

Lorin

As far back as I can remember, as early as 6 or 7, I masturbated. I was never sexually abused or raped; I did it because it felt good, it was soothing, and it helped me go to sleep. My mother saw me several times and had no idea how to respond, so she told me, "Don't do that, it's having sex with yourself!"

Fueling the Fire

At that age, I really had no idea what sex was, or why what I was doing was so bad. Eventually, the stimulation became an addiction to me, and as I grew older it developed a new purpose. As hormones raged in my early teens, the once (innocent) infantile masturbation or gratification disorder, developed into the self pleasure my mother once warned me about, and set the tone for my promiscuity. It was more than easy to find things to fantasize about during my "sessions of self pleasure." Between movies and the MTV and BET music channels, there were copious amounts of beautiful people engaging in sexual behavior right there in the middle of the day on my family's television. Coupled with severe insecurity, lust was the very thing to fuel my careless sex and licentious behavior.

I held onto my virginity until I was 17. Although I was not having sex prior to that, I did "fool around" with plenty of boys. When I finally did lose my virginity, the act of sex did not have any special meaning to it. Boys had become my favorite past time. My most enjoyed extracurricular activity was getting attention from the opposite sex. I was extremely insecure and horrified by my outward appearance, and years of verbal and physical abuse from my father left me wondering if anyone could ever love someone like me. My promiscuous behavior made me feel empowered, sexy, desired, special, beautiful, and most importantly loved. I felt that beyond a shadow of a doubt that I had nothing to offer anyone. Every fiber of my being rejoiced when I received attention. I needed it, craved it, and hungered for it. I became addicted to the affirmation of others, and I was infatuated with the idea of being someone's desire!

Enter Pornography...

I was introduced to pornography casually. The types of people I surrounded myself with indulged quite often with it. I would come across magazines every now and again, as well as movies. I had a good friend whose mother owned a huge collection of videos, and she would show them to me. I remember thinking to myself that the only explanation that they would excite me so much was that I was a lesbian or bisexual, because I was only attracted to the women. This thought made me uncomfortable at first, but I later found myself fully engaged in sexual activity with women. Pornography had completely ruined my perspective on the value of a woman, relationships, and the purpose of sex.

The Turning Point

A copy of the book Captivating had made it into my hands. The author described a romance with God, an unconditional love that gave me hope. It was the push I needed to break away from a particularly bad relationship and lifestyle. Not too long after ending that relationship once and for all, I met the man who is now my husband. I was still very broken, but God had begun to change my perspective on sex. I had not yet had any great revelation on the purpose of sex, but I began having convictions about promiscuity. I started going to church more frequently, however I withheld any great commitment to God. More than anything, I was curious if this "God" that seemed like a lost memory of my confusing childhood was really for me.

Pretty soon after meeting each other, we decided that we would get married. Nevertheless, I was living no differently than I had been. As I know now, marriage does not fix things. You will bring the problems you had as a single person and join them with your spouse's. We "dated" for two months before we were married. Two children later and about 5 years into our marriage, I still battled with an addiction to masturbation and pornography, the demons of my decisions, the soul ties I had formed, and the spiritual warfare I created with my past promiscuous behavior. I was consumed with depression, anxiety, and suicidal thoughts. I hit my breaking point when my "need for affirmation" mindset rose again while I was married. I did not want to be unfaithful to my husband; I refused to let my skeletons from my closet rise up and consume my marriage. I needed to settle and destroy this behavior, but how? It wasn't until I finally gave in and submitted my life, problems, and anguish, completely over to God that the healing finally began.

Becoming One with One Another and God

Accompanied with restoration, renewal, and a soul revival, God picked up the broken pieces and put them back together as soon as I lay them before Him. My husband has also since given his life to the Lord. Jesus is the center of my life, the foundation on which I grow, and God is the healer, restorer, comforter of our lives, and the foundation of our marriage, and family.

I can say honestly today, that I enjoy sex with my husband on a completely different level. I understand the purpose of sex finally, not being for self pleasure but, as an establishment of a blood covenant between a groom and his bride, the act of coming together, being unified, more close to one another than to anything else. When two become one, a life is established, a life of togetherness, trust, holiness, purity, righteousness, and unity. It is amazing, I feel united with him. It is very obviously a spiritual-God-ordained gift to be shared between a husband and a wife. It is only by the grace of God that I am freed from the many strongholds I formed while disregarding the discomfort of the Holy Spirit in my choice making. I strongly urge any young woman today to abstain from sex, stay pure, live a lifestyle that is pleasing to God, separate yourself from earthly mindsets, and do not become accustomed to the culture of secularism.

Sex is more than a big deal. God can indeed restore your purity, but there is no need to be broken when you can avoid it all together. Spend your time as a single falling in love with Jesus and pursuing his plan for your life. The person you give your heart (and virginity) to should be so sold out to Jesus that he demands Christ is your first love too!

PART THREE:
HOW TO BREAK FREE

Shelley Hitz

Are you ready to be free? If you have read this far (or skipped forward to this section) you are most likely looking for answers on how to break free from an addiction to pornography and/or masturbation. First of all, I want to remind you that you are not alone. When I was in the midst of my struggle with pornography and masturbation, I thought I was the <u>only</u> Christian woman to ever struggle with this particular sin, and I felt as if there was something inherently wrong with me. However, these are lies that the enemy, Satan, uses to keep us in bondage to our sin and trapped in shame.

Secondly, I want to remind you that we are saved by God's grace alone. It is only by His grace we are saved from our sin, including the sin of pornography. There is nothing we can do in our own strength to earn His grace. It is there for all of us – no matter what we have done, where we have been or what has been done to us. Each one of us can have a fresh start today and be free from the shame and regret of our past.

I am so thankful that Jesus had the victory in my life. He has given me freedom from pornography and He wants to do the same for you. Isaiah 61:1 says, "The Spirit of the Sovereign Lord is on me, because the Lord has anointed me to proclaim good news to the poor. He has sent me to bind up the brokenhearted, to proclaim freedom for the captives and release from darkness for the prisoners."

And yet, your path to freedom may not look exactly like mine. We are all uniquely created with different backgrounds and life circumstances. Therefore, I do not believe there is just one step-by-step system to break free from pornography. I wish I had an "easy button" to give to you right now, but I do not.

However, in this section I am going to share with you a list of practical steps you can apply to your life to break free from pornography. Some of these steps can be applied to other addictions in your life, whereas others will be related specifically to pornography. Please do not feel like you need to do every single step that I share with you in this section. Instead, I encourage you to pray and ask God for wisdom. Ask Him to show you which specific steps you should take on your path to freedom, and then, take that first step.

"A journey of a thousand miles begins with a single step."

~Lao-tzu

Chapter 10
The First Step Is Forgiveness

One of the first steps that we need to take with any sin in our lives is forgiveness. It is not just a matter of good intentions and wanting to do better, but of depending on Christ's forgiveness to restore our purity and wash us clean again.

There was once a newspaper that reported the top phrases people love to hear. The number one phrase was "I love you." Number two was "dinner is served," and number three was "I forgive you."

Forgiveness. Is. Powerful.

I am passionate about sharing on this topic of forgiveness. Why? Well, just about every major turning point in my life spiritually has started with forgiveness. It has been a powerful catalyst in my life for spiritual growth and healing from wounds of the past.

What Makes Forgiveness So Powerful?

Have you ever been forgiven a debt that you owed to someone else? It feels good to not have to pay that money back, does it not? Now, imagine that someone came to you today and said that mortgage, school loans and/or credit card debt has been forgiven. It has been erased and you no longer have to pay those bills. Would you be happy? You bet! Personally, I would be throwing a big party if my mortgage was paid off today.

And so we see that forgiveness is powerful.

The Weight of Unforgiveness

I heard an illustration once about unforgiveness that I will never forget. Imagine that unforgiveness is like carrying a dead corpse around on your back, "piggy back." You carry that weight around everywhere you go.

Do you know what would happen to you physically from carrying a dead person around on your back? It is pretty gross, actually. As the dead corpse continues to rot and decay, it would eventually cause your healthy tissue to rot and decay as well. Over time, it would literally begin to "eat away" at you.

That is the picture of unforgiveness. Over time, unforgiveness, bitterness, and resentment will begin to eat away at us emotionally and spiritually.

The longer you carry it, the heavier it becomes. Just like carrying a backpack around with you on a long hike, that gets heavier with each mile you walk, unforgiveness becomes a heavy weight emotionally and spiritually with each passing day.

What Does the Bible Say about Unforgiveness?

I do not want to assume that you know what the Bible says about unforgiveness, so let us take a look at a couple of verses.

For if you forgive men when they sin against you, your heavenly Father will also forgive you. But if you do not forgive men their sins, your Father will not forgive your sins.

Matthew 6:14-15

If you have anything against anyone, forgive him and let it drop (leave it, let it go) in order that your Father who is in heaven may also forgive you your [own] failings and shortcomings and let them drop. But if you do not forgive, neither will your Father in heaven forgive your failings and shortcomings.

Mark 11:25-26 (AMP)

I like the way the Amplified version puts it. *Let it drop (leave it, let it go).* I picture myself letting go of the weight of unforgiveness I have been carrying around for all these years; letting it drop into the hands of Jesus.

The Forgiveness Cross

An illustration that has helped me to walk through the process of forgiveness in my life is the forgiveness cross. It represents three different parts of forgiveness, as you can see below.

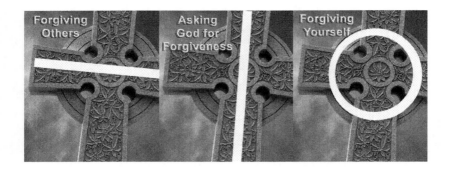

1. Forgiving Others
2. Asking God for Forgiveness
3. Forgiving Yourself

I realized in my own journey that there were people I needed to forgive…people who had sexually abused me. I also needed to ask God for His forgiveness of my sin against Him, and finally, I needed to forgive myself.

Many times, forgiving ourselves is the hardest part. I remember after Christ set me free from my struggle with pornography, I was having difficulty forgiving myself. I had forgiven others, I had repented and asked God's forgiveness, and I had repented and changed directions. God was empowering me to live differently and I was making good decisions.

Yet, there was this regret that lingered.

You see, I was a Christian when I made these mistakes. I knew better, and I just couldn't allow myself to forget it. I was living in regret.

It was as if Satan would taunt me and remind me of all my failures and mistakes of the past.

"Shelley, you do not deserve to be in ministry. Look how you failed God. You'll just fail Him again. Look at those years you wasted in self-centeredness and pride. You'll never know what impact you could have had for Christ if you would have just been obedient to God in the first place. You are nothing but a failure."

And on and on it went. I was tortured by these thoughts of regret.

One day I was driving down the road and Matthew West's song "History" came on the radio. The song talks about the mistakes, the regrets, and the moments we wish we could take back. Then it says, "Yesterday is history and history is miles away, so leave it all behind you. Let it always remind you of the day that Love made history."

I distinctly sensed God saying to me in my heart, "Shelley, you have forgiven others, but you cannot forgive yourself. It is time to let go of this regret and forgive yourself."

I had to pull over to the side of the road because I was crying so hard. It was true. I needed to forgive myself. As I did, a weight was lifted off of me. I was forgiven and I could move on.

That day was a turning point for me.

Application:

1. Go through the steps of the forgiveness cross.

I encourage you to walk through these steps of forgiveness as God leads you. Ask Him if there is still anyone that you need to forgive in your life, ask God for His forgiveness and then take the necessary step of forgiving yourself.

And before you move on to the next chapter in this book, the most critical element of this journey to freedom is to know where you stand with Jesus. Who is Jesus to you? If you are unsure, I encourage you to read what I have written for you on the link below, before moving forward in this book. The rest of this book hinges upon knowing Jesus and having a relationship with Him. Therefore, it is really important for you to read this first here:

www.bodyandsoulpublishing.com/jesus

2. Watch this video

In a video presentation titled, "The Power of Forgiveness," I share my own battle with forgiving my grandma's murderer as well as forgiving myself for my regrets of the past. You will also hear from my dad who shares how he was able to forgive his assailant that left him in a coma for almost 8 weeks with a traumatic brain injury. Watch this powerful presentation at:

www.christianspeakers.tv/forgiveness

3. Go deeper.

If you want to go deeper on this topic of forgiveness, I encourage you to read our books below:

The Forgiveness Formula: Finding Lasting Freedom in Christ

Unshackled and Free: True Stories of Forgiveness

Chapter 11
The Key Is Surrender

I still vividly remember my internal struggle with pornography. For a season, I enjoyed the temporary satisfaction that came with indulging in porn. However, that feeling of pleasure did not last forever. Eventually, I felt trapped and I desperately wanted out.

I finally reached a breaking point, and I was desperate.

An Illustration God Gave Me

Have you ever watched a football game and noticed what happens to the winning football coach after a major victory? Many times you will see several of the team members dump a big cooler of ice water over the coach's head.

That is the picture God gave me of what happened in my life. It was as if God, through the conviction of His Holy Spirit, poured a big cooler of ice water over my head.

Suddenly I woke up to the reality of my sin.

I knew that if I continued in this cycle of pornography and masturbation, it would lead to destruction, eventually destroying my spiritual life and my marriage. I also knew I could not "get better" on my own, so after much struggle, I finally surrendered to Christ.

There is nothing magical about this step of surrender. It is simply a willingness to allow Christ full access into your heart and life…and a willingness to change.

I have counseled women struggling with pornography that have felt the conviction of the Holy Spirit. They have told me they want to change, but, after talking in depth with them, I realized that even though they felt the conviction of their sin, they were not yet willing to fully surrender.

How About You?

Are you desperate enough to allow God to do His work in your life? It may be painful at first, but it will be worth it. Believe me on this one!

God often speaks to me in illustrations and pictures. The picture I see is of a surgeon cutting open a patient's abdomen in order to remove a big cancerous tumor in the patient's stomach. Yes, the surgeon is causing more pain to the patient by cutting them open, but in the end, the surgeon is actually saving the patient's life by removing this cancerous tumor hidden within their body.

As I found out in my life, pornography is a "cancer" to the soul that can lead to spiritual death.

Are you ready for surgery?

Application:

1. Prayer of Surrender

Pray a prayer of surrender to Christ asking Him to empower you to change. You can pray through Psalm 51, which is a prayer of repentance from David after he sinned sexually in an adulterous affair with Bathsheba. Or you can pray something like this,

Lord, I want to be free from anything that weighs me down and the sin that so easily entangles (Hebrews 12:1-2). I surrender to You my heart, mind and will and ask that You lead me through this this journey to healing and freedom. Help me to be willing to deal with the issues of my past that are hindering my spiritual growth. I acknowledge Your power to overcome sin and to help me do what I cannot do myself. Empower me to change through your Holy Spirit. Amen.

Chapter 12
Have You Opened the Door to the Enemy?

Then, it is time to close it!

You might have grown up with parents who told you not to open the door of your house to strangers. Do you remember what your parents said the stranger might have to entice you to open the door? Something like candy or a fun toy, right? And yet they probably told you the stranger might have motives to harm you. Your parents were simply trying to protect you from harm.

Our enemy is like that stranger. The Bible says in John 10:10 that Satan has come to "steal, kill, and destroy" us. He comes with enticing gifts that are fun and pleasurable, but deep down his motives are to harm us and draw us away from our relationship with Jesus.

If You Have Opened the Door to Satan, How Do You Close It?

How do you close the door that has been opened to sexual strongholds in your life?

1. First, you must recognize your sin.

2. Then, go back to the place, where by your sin, you opened your heart to the influence of Satan and his demons. Close the door by confessing your sin to Jesus.

3. Claim Jesus' promise in I John 1:7-9 to cleanse you and forgive you. He is able to turn your darkness into light.

4. Finally, it is time to repent, turn from the sin in your life, and ask Jesus to empower you to change.

One of the ways the "door" to sexual strongholds was opened in my life was through an instance of sexual abuse that happened when I was in eighth grade and then another sexual encounter with a boyfriend in high school. God took me through the process of forgiving both of them as well as asking God's forgiveness for my part in it. Finally, I needed to forgive myself. It was time to close the door that was opened in my life!

Generational Patterns

Another way the "door" to sexual sin can be opened in our lives is from generational patterns and strongholds. Maybe there is a history of sexual sin in your family. There could be certain patterns that you may have been taught growing up or were exposed to at an early age in regards to sexuality.

In my family, there was a history of sexual sin. Honestly, I did not think it was a big deal and did not believe it impacted me. However, one day I went through a prayer to break any sexual strongholds that were created by my ancestors and to forgive them for anything they passed along to me. I also asked God's forgiveness and forgave myself for participating in this sin. I can't fully explain it, but I literally felt something lift from me that day in the spiritual realm. It was one more "door" that God closed in my life in regards to sexual sin.

We Are in a Spiritual Battle

The Bible is very clear that we are in the midst of a spiritual battle. Ephesians 6:12 says, "For we do not wrestle against flesh and blood, but against principalities, against powers, against the rulers of the darkness of this age, against spiritual hosts of wickedness."

According to Barna research, 40% of Christians do not believe the Devil exists. However, even if you do not believe in the devil, you most likely believe in evil. [1]

And what is evil? Evil is live spelled backwards. So, you can think of evil as this…evil is when we live life backwards.

Jesus Came to Undo the Works of Satan

Here are just a few reminders that Jesus came to undo the works of Satan in our lives.

That through death [Jesus] might destroy him who had the power of death, that is, the devil.

Hebrews 2:14

The reason the Son of God (Jesus) appeared was to destroy the devil's work.

1 John 3:8b

And having disarmed the powers and authorities, [Jesus] made a public spectacle of them triumphing over them by the cross.

Colossians 2:15

You are of God...and have overcome them, because He who is in you is greater than he who is in the world.

1 John 4:4

Application:

1. Close the door.

It is time to close the door to Satan in your life. Go through steps one through four above as God leads you. Ask Him to reveal specific times and places that the door to sexual strongholds was opened in your life.

2. Go through "Steps to Freedom"

I recommend you take this step even further by going through Neil Anderson's, "Steps to Freedom in Christ." Our ministry has been given permission to use this valuable resource with those we counsel and minister to within our ministry. Contact us here to get more information and download this powerful guide here:

www.bodyandsoulpublishing.com/freedom

3. Put on the armor of God each day

It is important to realize that we are in a spiritual battle. And to prepare, the Bible tells us in Ephesians 6 that we are to put on our spiritual armor. I recommend praying through Ephesians 6:10-20 and asking God to protect you with His armor each morning before you begin your day. You can read the warrior's prayer and download an audio version based on these scriptures by Dr. David Jeremiah here:

www.bodyandsoulpublishing.com/warrior

Chapter 13
Accountability: One Key to Breaking Free

What is accountability? Accountability is where you ask someone you trust to meet with you regularly to pray together and to ask you the hard questions.

As an author, I know some authors that have writing accountability partners. They hold each other accountable to continue writing. Many times this means they set specific goals for themselves as far as how many words they will write, and so on.

Other people have accountability partners for losing weight. I know some people that go to meetings each week where they have to "weigh in." This accountability helps them stay consistent with healthy eating habits and exercise, when they would otherwise give up.

During my struggle with pornography, I found that having an accountability partner was one of the main things God used in my life to help set me free.

A Biblical Illustration of Accountability

When I think of accountability, I think of a certain story about Moses in the Bible when the Israelites went to battle against

72

the Amalekites. This story can be found in Exodus 17:8-12 as follows:

Now Amalek came and fought with Israel in Rephidim. And Moses said to Joshua, 'Choose us some men and go out, fight with Amalek. Tomorrow I will stand on the top of the hill with the rod of God in my hand.'

So Joshua did as Moses said to him, and fought with Amalek. And Moses, Aaron, and Hur went up to the top of the hill. And so it was, when Moses held up his hand, that Israel prevailed; and when he let down his hand, Amalek prevailed.

But Moses' hands became heavy; so they took a stone and put it under him, and he sat on it. **And Aaron and Hur supported his hands, one on one side, and the other on the other side;** *and his hands were steady until the going down of the sun. So Joshua defeated Amalek and his people with the edge of the sword.*

To summarize, the Israelites had victory in the battle when Moses held up his hands. However, during the middle of the battle, he got tired. But instead of giving into defeat, Aaron and Hur came alongside him and supported his hands until the victory was won.

This is such a vivid illustration of what I believe happens to us as Christians in the spiritual battles we face each day. Although we are given the empowerment of the Holy Spirit, we are still human and sometimes get battle weary. And that is when we need other Christians in our lives to help support us, so we can have the victory over sin in our lives.

We Need Each Other

As a Christian, we are part of the body of Christ and we need each other. Just like each part of our physical body is dependent on the other, as Christians we are to be dependent on one another. However, in our culture, instead of embracing the community of believers around us, we often live independent lives from each other in isolation.

Isolation is exactly where Satan wants us. When we are isolated, we are more vulnerable to his attacks. Just like a sheep that gets isolated from the herd is more vulnerable to attacks from its predators, coyotes and wolves, we are also more vulnerable to spiritual attacks when we live in isolation from other believers.

We may think we can handle our sin on our own, but many times God wants us to humble ourselves and ask for help.

James 5:17 says, "Therefore confess your sins to each other and pray for each other so that you may be healed. The prayer of a righteous person is powerful and effective."

Notice that it says you are to confess your sins to each other, so that you may be healed. Do you want to be healed? If so, I recommend that you ask God to help you lay down your pride, so that you can share your struggle with someone else and receive the prayer support you need.

It Is Difficult to Confess Our Sins to Each Other

I have to admit it was difficult for me to share my struggle with the sin of pornography with others. This sin, more than others, tends to be very shame-based. Did you know that there is a difference between true guilt and shame? True guilt is the conviction of the Holy Spirit that we have sinned and done something wrong. True guilt leads to repentance, healing and freedom. However, shame is the voice inside your mind that says, "I am a bad person. I cannot believe I am doing this. I cannot let anyone know how depraved I have become. I have to keep this a secret." The voice of shame often keeps us from reaching out to ask someone to be our accountability partner. Ask God for healing from the shame in your life. Then, ask Him to give you the strength you need to share your sin with an accountability partner.

Pornography is a sin that is often done in secret. Therefore, no one else knows about it unless you tell them or unless they catch you in the act. The more secretive a sin is, the more power it holds over a person.

Think about mold...it grows strongest in the darkness. But when you bring mold out of the darkness and into the light, it dies.

And often, something similar happens in our spiritual lives with sin. When we bring our sin out into the light by confessing it to another believer, the power that sin has over us weakens. I know this has been true for me in my life.

And unfortunately, the sin of pornography is not often "brought out into the light" in many churches today. Think about it. How many sermons have you heard preached about pornography from your pastor? Probably not very many. That is because it is not a topic often mentioned in the Church. It is uncomfortable to discuss, so many times, we simply avoid it.

Some women have confided in me that they are hesitant to share about their struggle with someone in the Church because they are afraid they will be judged and looked down upon. The important part is to pray and ask God to provide you with an accountability partner you can trust, someone who will show you love and grace and yet still ask you the hard questions.

Finding an Accountability Partner You Can Trust

How do you know if you can trust someone? Watch their lives.

For example, say you have a friend that you would like to ask to be your accountability partner. Look back on your friendship with that person. Does your friend often share with you personal information from other peoples' lives? If so, then realize that they may also share personal information that you have told them in confidence with others.

Proverbs 20:19 says, "A gossip betrays a confidence; so avoid anyone who talks too much."

That is good advice. When I look for an accountability partner, I look for someone that does not gossip about others to me. I also look for someone who is strong in their faith in Christ. If someone is not a believer or is not strong in their faith, they may give me advice or counsel that is not godly, not biblical and ultimately not helpful to me.

Trust God to Provide Someone for You

When I talk to women and teen girls about finding an accountability partner, often it comes with resistance. Many times I hear excuses like, "There is no one in my life to be my accountability partner," or "Shelley, you just do not understand. There is no one I can trust in my life."

I realize there is some validity to their responses. However, I have also been in a similar place in my life and God has proven to me over and over that He can provide exactly what I need, when I need it.

During the time when I struggled with pornography, my best friend from high school lived in the same town with me. Shortly after that, she moved thousands of miles away, but God provided her friendship, accountability and prayers when I needed it the most. She was someone I could trust and I knew would respond to me with grace and love, but would also ask me the hard questions, which she did.

There were only about three or four people in all, including my counselor and my husband that knew I was struggling with this sin at that time. I did not broadcast it to the world. Do not think that you need to tell everyone. I recommend only sharing it with a few people you can trust, possibly your pastor, your spouse, a parent, a close friend, etc.

I think about it like this. One of my friends once shared with me that when she is in the middle of a struggle, she calls it a "moan-ey". However, when God brings her to the other side of her struggle and has given her freedom and healing, she then calls it a "testimony," so when you are in the middle of your "moan-ey," I recommend only telling a few trusted people. But, once you have a testimony, then you can share it with more people as God leads you.

And that is what I am doing in this book. I am now sharing my testimony, the freedom and healing that Christ has given me to encourage others. Revelation 12:11 says that we overcome our enemy Satan as we share our testimony. "They triumphed over [Satan] by the blood of the Lamb (Jesus) and by the word of their testimony."

So there is a time and a place to share your testimony, but now is not the time.

Application

1. Identify an accountability partner

I encourage you to pray about who you should ask to be your accountability partner. Once you have identified someone, take the step to ask them to start meeting with you on a regular basis. Do it! Do not delay. This is an important step.

If no one comes to mind, ask God to provide an accountability partner for you, and many times He will. Also, realize that there are seasons in our lives that God may have us walk through something with Him alone, so try not to get stuck at this step. Even if you currently do not have anyone in your life to meet with, continue through the other steps until you have freedom from pornography in your life.

2. Start meeting together

In the past, when I was struggling with pornography, I met with my accountability partner on a weekly basis for prayer and accountability. But in another season of my life, I met with an accountability partner on a monthly basis. You know yourself and what will work best for you and your schedule. The important thing is to be <u>consistent</u> in meeting together on a regular basis.

3. Pray together and ask the hard questions

I recommend praying together each time you meet, but I also think it is important to have your accountability partner ask you the hard questions. Your questions may be slightly different than mine, but here are some sample questions you can use.

- How has your spiritual life been? Have you prayed, sincerely, and been reading God's Word?

- Have you viewed any pornographic images since we last met, intentionally or unintentionally?

- Have you acted out in any way since we last met? If so, how, and what steps will you take to avoid doing so in the future?

- Have you done anything since we last met that you are ashamed of?

- Have you lied to me today in any of your answers?

- How can I pray for you today?

Chapter 14
Using Computer Filters and Software

An obvious recommendation for anyone struggling with pornography is to use computer filters and software. It is just one way to help you in your desire to be free. However, pornography is an internal struggle that stems from your heart. Jesus said in Matthew 5:28, "But I say to you that whoever looks at a woman to lust for her has already committed adultery with her in his heart." The point he was making is that adultery is not just a physical act, but also about our thoughts. And so if you only set up external boundaries, like computer filters and software, you are not likely to find lasting freedom.

However, my husband and I have found that using computer filters and software have been helpful to us as we desire to stay free from pornography. And so I will share a few options with you in the list below. Some we have personally used, and some we have not. I encourage you to do some of your own research as well to decide which would be best for you.

Free Software

X3watch Free

If your budget is tight, you can still download the free version of X3watch software on your PC or Mac. We have used both the free and pro versions of this software in the past. You can identify three accountability partners that will receive a report of questionable websites you have visited. When we were using this software, my husband asked my mom to be one of these three people. He said, "There's nothing like knowing your mother-in-law will be seeing your browsing report to keep you on the straight and narrow." You could also ask your pastor, spouse and accountability partner to receive these reports.

Download the free version here:
www.bodyandsoulpublishing.com/x3watchfree

Paid Software

Covenant Eyes

Covenant Eyes is also a well-known and popular accountability and filtering software. One thing that sets them apart is that accountability for your mobile devices (iPhone®, iPod Touch®, and iPad®, and web and app monitoring for all Android™ phones and tablets) is included with no additional cost when you sign up for internet accountability.

According to the Covenant Eyes website, "nearly one in five searches made from mobile devices are for pornography" and so having this additional feature is valuable to you.

Here are the current costs for Covenant Eyes:

First username
Accountability only: $8.99/mo.
Filtering only: $4.99/mo.
Both: $10.49/mo.

Each additional username
Accountability only: $2.00/mo.
Filtering only: $1.50/mo.
Both: $3.50/mo.

Get started with Covenant Eyes here:
www.bodyandsoulpublishing.com/covenanteyes

X3watch Pro

X3watch also has a pro version that has a monthly fee. At the time of writing this, the fee is $7 per month and offers you these additional features:

- Flag or Block websites
- Monitor/Block Video & P2P?
- Text message alerts
- Unlimited accountability partners
- Free technical support by phone, email or online helpdesk
- Works on 10 computers

Download the paid version here:
www.bodyandsoulpublishing.com/x3watchpro

X3watch for Mobile Devices

X3watch also offers apps for your mobile devices. They are currently $6.99 and you can find out more information about them here:

iPhone/iPad:
www.bodyandsoulpublishing.com/x3watchiphone

Android:
www.bodyandsoulpublishing.com/x3watchandroid

Safe Eyes

Safe Eyes is Mac, PC, and iOS compatible software that protects your family from harmful content and other dangers on the internet.

Safe Eyes Software Includes:

- Content Controls - Flexible content control allows you to select the types of websites and content that are appropriate.
- Program Controls - Control Instant Messengers, iTunes, P2P File Sharing, and other harmful programs.
- Time Controls - Control the amount of time spent online, and the times when the internet is available.
- Usage Logging - Create and review logs of websites visited, programs used on the Internet, and Instant Messaging Chats.

- Usage Alerts - Be notified instantly via email, text message, or phone call when someone visits inappropriate websites.

Safe Eyes for PC/Mac is $49.95/year for 3 licenses (which equals $4.16/month)

Safe Eyes mobile app for iOS is $14.99

Get started with Safe Eyes here:
www.bodyandsoulpublishing.com/safeeyes

SafeCell

SafeCell's Mobile provides controls by:

- Monitoring your mobile phone use and sending instant alerts if you receives unapproved email, text messages, photos or phone calls.
- Monitoring and blocking websites.
- Blocking applications
- Setting time restrictions for your phone usage.

Try SafeCell for 30 day free, then $9.95/month:
www.bodyandsoulpublishing.com/safecell

Application

1. Choose your accountability and internet filter software.

In this day and age it is important to have software not only for your computer, but also your mobile devices. The three most popular are Covenant Eyes, X3watch and Safe Eyes. Decide which you will use for your computer and each of your mobile devices.

2. Get started using the software

Download your software of choice and get started using it right away. You have no excuse as there is even a free option. This extra layer of protection is just one tool God can use in your life as you break free from an addiction to pornography.

Chapter 15
Identify the Triggers

When I was in counseling during my struggle with pornography, the counselor asked me to identify any consistent triggers that would cause me to give in to the temptation of pornography and/or masturbation.

What Are Triggers?

When I think about the word, trigger, I automatically think of a gun. A gun can sit in your house for months, even years, fully loaded, and never harm someone. However, the moment the trigger is pulled, that is when the damage is done. In the same way, it is not a sin to be tempted to lust or look at pornography. The sin comes when we act upon the temptation, either in our mind or physically.

Many times there are "triggers" that can cause an automatic reaction within us, like the "snowball" effect. Once you get the snowball rolling down a hill, it is difficult to stop. And I know that this was the case for me with pornography and certain triggers.

It Is Different for Everyone

What triggers each of us to sin will be different for everyone, but for me, one of my triggers was looking at the DVD covers in our local movie rental store. Have you looked at the DVD covers lately? Unfortunately there are a lot of them with very seductive looking images. Many times I would go to our movie rental store, see these images, and be triggered to go searching for pornography online later. Once I realized this was a consistent trigger for me, I stopped going to the movie rental store. With the technology available to us now, we now rent our movies online at locations like iTunes or Amazon instead of going in person to the movie rental store. This was just one way I was able to eliminate a trigger in my life.

Another trigger for me was watching movies and music videos with a lot of sensuality in them. And unfortunately it did not take much for me to be triggered. Therefore I stopped listening to certain music, stopped watching music videos online, and started reading online reviews of the movies before we watched them. If the review said there was going to be nudity, sensuality or sex scenes in the movie, then I avoided watching it...even if it was a Blockbuster "must see" movie.

For movie reviews, we use the Plugged-in Online website, a ministry of Focus on the Family: http://www.pluggedin.com. You can also get reviews of music and video games at this website as well.

The Narrow Path

Often the path to freedom is steep and difficult. I have been on hiking trails that were very difficult to climb. But it never fails, once I get to the top of the mountain I am so glad that I pushed through the pain and difficulty and did not give up.

The picture below is from the South Sister Mountain in Oregon. Hiking to the summit was one of the most difficult things I have ever done, but the view of ten other mountains from the top is one I will never forget.

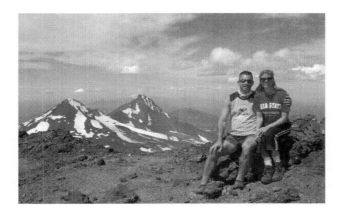

Matthew 7:13-14 says, "Enter by the narrow gate; for wide is the gate and broad is the way that leads to destruction, and there are many who go in by it. Because narrow is the gate and difficult is the way which leads to life, and there are few who find it."

I will admit that at times it has been very difficult to make the decision to limit our media consumption. We are not trying to be legalistic and follow certain "rules" by limiting our music and movie choices; we do this because we want to stay free and experience true life. We have chosen this path because we do not want to be triggered into a struggle from the past.

Application

1. Write out your triggers

Sit down and write out any consistent triggers in your life regarding pornography and/or masturbation.   If nothing comes to mind, keep a journal for 1-2 weeks and write out what you did, where you were or what you were doing prior to watching pornography. Look at your journal and see if there are any consistent triggers.

Some triggers are common to all of us.   One acronym I learned from my mom, who is a Christian counselor, is H.A.L.T.   It stands for Hungry, Angry, Lonely or Tired. These are four common triggers that can leave us vulnerable to temptation, especially when you are experiencing more than one of them at a time. So be aware that you may be more vulnerable to temptation when you are hungry, angry, lonely and/or tired.

I also used a calendar to help me identify my triggers. Find out more and see an example of one of my calendars from June of 2000 when I was still struggling with pornography here:

www.bodyandsoulpublishing.com/calendar

2. Ask God for wisdom

Next, pray and ask God for wisdom on how to avoid and overcome these triggers.   Write out any ideas that come to mind in your journal.

3. Finally, take action.

Do what you can to eliminate or avoid the consistent triggers you identified as much as possible. I realize that you still need to live in our culture and will not be able to eliminate every trigger, but there will be some that you can avoid that will make a huge difference to help you be free and stay free.

Note: I know that for some of the women and teen girls I counsel, one of their main triggers is their smartphone or mobile device. There are filters available for these devices, but if it is something that is consistently causing you to fall in this area of temptation, ask yourself if you are willing to do something radical in order to be free. Is your freedom from this sin worth it?

If so, you may need to consider taking some radical steps.

I have heard people say that when they would feeling the urge to watch pornography and/or masturbate, they would read a chapter of the gospels. If they still felt the urge, they would read another chapter. Another person said that every time they were tempted with sexual sin, they would fast from food for at least one meal and devote that time to prayer. They said the more they fasted and prayed, the less the temptations came. Eventually the enemy will give up as he realizes the temptation is only drawing you closer to Christ instead of further away.

Another example of a radical step is to get a new phone without a data plan or deactivate the internet access on your device (i.e iPad, tablet). I know it may sound impossible to live without internet access on your mobile devices, but nothing is impossible for God (Luke 1:37).

For a season of time, I had my husband put a password on our computer that only he had access to. That way, I could only use our computer when he was home. If your job requires you to have access to the internet, you may choose to use the internet in a public place with accountability and filtering software on all of your computers and devices.

I know these suggestions may sound radical to you, but think about this: let's say you see a child who is running after his ball into the street in front of a semi-truck. You see him headed for danger and realize that his parents are too far away to do anything about it, so you race toward the child, and grab him away from the street as fast as you can. Unfortunately, in doing so, you not only save the child's life but you also dislocate both of his shoulders and cause deep gashes in both of his legs. Do you think this child's parents are going to scream at you in anger saying, "Why did you do that? Don't you see how much you have hurt my child!?!" No, I do not think that will be their reaction at all. We know that any right-minded parent is going to realize that you just saved their child's life. You will be a hero to that family. And they will probably thank you over and over again throughout the years for saving the life of their child.

I see an addiction to pornography in a similar way. You may get some gashes and experience some pain along your path to freedom, but in the process, you will be saved from a gradual spiritual death. And believe me, I know from personal experience that the temporary pain you will experience as you eliminate these triggers in your life, far outweighs the pain and consequences of continuing down the same destructive path of a pornography addiction.   It is time to do the hard things and hike up the narrow path that leads to LIFE.

Chapter 16
The Importance of a Father's Love
And What to Do If You Grew up Lacking It

You will often hear someone say, "She's Daddy's little girl." Deep down, I think being "Daddy's little girl" is something we girls long for...to be loved, cherished and treasured by our fathers.

However, the reality is that many of us grew up without the stability, security and protection of a loving father. Instead, our fathers may have been distant emotionally, absent from the home, too busy working, abusive or neglectful, and we may have left childhood feeling unloved by our dads for one reason or another. This can then leave us looking for ways to fill that longing, and sometimes we use pornography as a coping mechanism.

Fathers Will Have an Impact on Their Daughter's Life...

...either positively or negatively.

Don't get me wrong. A mother's nurturing love is essential. We need the love from both our mother and our father, but our dads have a different impact on us.

- They teach us how to interact with guys.

- They teach us how a guy should treat a girl.
- They are the first man in our lives that has the opportunity to affirm our beauty and teach us that our beauty goes beyond skin deep.
- They model how a husband should treat his wife.
- And so forth.

Did you feel secure in your father's love and protection growing up? Did you know that he had your best interests in mind? Did your dad affirm your beauty and worth and show you respect?

Unfortunately, many girls do not receive affirmation and love from their fathers; therefore it is easy to go looking for it somewhere else.

The Impact on Our Relationship with God

Sometimes we end up projecting our feelings about our earthly father onto our heavenly Father. If we feel like our earthy father is distant emotionally from us, we may assume that our heavenly Father is the same. If our earthly father has disappointed us and let us down, we may think that our heavenly Father will disappoint us as well. If our earthly father wasn't safe for us, but instead was abusive, we may have a difficult time trusting our heavenly Father to be a safe haven for us.

Do you see how this can happen?

I know it did for me. And I had to realize that God is not like my dad. He won't let me down or disappoint me. I had to be reminded of the character of God, my heavenly Father, through His Word, the Bible. It shows over and over that God is loving, trustworthy, and has my best interests in mind.

I had to slowly begin to change the way I saw God, and you may have to do that as well.

You Can Have a Father That Loves You Completely

Are you longing for someone to love you completely and unconditionally? Before you try to find that love "in all the wrong places" like I did, realize that you can find that love in your heavenly Father. It may be hard for you to accept His love right now. You may not feel very love-able, or you may doubt that God really cares for you.

It is okay to wrestle with those feelings. You are on a journey, a journey of healing. Will you allow God to love you and satisfy all your deepest longings? Will you let go of your past and forgive your earthly father for the ways he didn't provide that love for you?

Your heavenly Father is waiting for you. He says, "Come near to me and I will come near to you" (James 4:8). He offers to love you completely as a Father should (Ephesians 3:19), and nothing can separate you from His love (Romans 8:35-39)

Will you accept His invitation?

Application

1. Reflect on your relationship with your earthly father

Take time to reflect on your relationship with your earthly father. Is there anything you need to bring to God right now? It could be feelings of hurt, abandonment, rejection, unforgiveness, etc. Pray and ask God to bring healing in your heart.

2. Reflect on your relationship with your heavenly Father

Now reflect on your relationship with your heavenly Father. Does He seem close to you or distant? Do you find yourself projecting your relationship with your earthly father onto God?

Pray and ask God to bring healing to any distorted view of God that you may have. Realize that He is the only man in your life who will never leave you, disappoint you or hurt you.

Chapter 17
When You Feel Broken Hearted

All of us have been hurt at some time in our lives and are in need of emotional healing. Whether it has been a bad break-up, parents' divorce, death in the family, abuse, rejection from friends....we've all been there at one time or another.

There have been several times in my life when I was in need of some emotional healing. I want to share with you some of the things that helped me through some pretty difficult times (death in the family, parents' divorce, sexual abuse, etc.).

I wish there were quick and easy emotional healing methods I could share with you that would give you instant healing. I do believe that God has the power to heal us instantly, but most of the time He allows us to heal slowly.

John Eldredge says, "If you wanted to learn how to heal the blind and you thought that following Christ around and watching how he did it would make things clear, you'd wind up pretty frustrated. He never does it the same way twice. He spits on one guy; for another, he spits on the ground and makes mud and puts that on his eyes. To a third he simply speaks, a fourth he touches, and for a fifth he kicks out a demon.

There are no formulas with God. The way in which God heals our wounds is a deeply personal process. He is a person and He insists on working personally.

For some, it comes in a moment of divine touch. For others, it takes place over time and through the help of another, maybe several others."[1]

Where Do You Start?

Unfortunately, I can't tell you exactly what to do. I wish I could. But, everyone is different and responds differently. Ultimately, you will need to get in touch with God and ask Him for wisdom on where to start.

James 1:5-8 says, "If anyone lacks wisdom, (she) should ask God, who gives generously to all without finding fault. But when (she) asks, (she) must believe and not doubt, because (she) who doubts is like a wave of the sea, blown and tossed by the wind. That (girl) should not think (she) will receive anything from the Lord; (she) is a double-minded (girl), unstable in all (she) does." (changed to feminine)

Healing Is Possible

Whatever you are going through, it is important to know that Jesus has the power to heal you.

Jesus went throughout Galilee, teaching in their synagogues, preaching the good news of the kingdom, and healing every disease and sickness among the people.

Matthew 4:23

And the people all tried to touch him, because power was coming from him and healing them all.

Luke 6:19

He welcomed them and spoke to them about the kingdom of God, and healed those who needed healing.

Luke 9:11

Jesus said to him, 'I will go and heal him.'

Matthew 8:7

When evening came, many who were demon-possessed were brought to him, and he drove out the spirits with a word and healed all the sick.

Matthew 8:16

A bruised reed he will not break, and a smoldering wick he will not snuff out.

Matthew 12:20

The Spirit of the Lord is upon me, because he hath anointed me to preach the gospel to the poor; he hath sent me to heal the brokenhearted, to preach deliverance to the captives, and recovering of sight to the blind, to set at liberty them that are bruised, to preach the acceptable year of the Lord.

Luke 4:18-19

My Broken Heart Restored...

I shared in an earlier chapter that I experienced an incident of sexual abuse when I was in eighth grade. I did not recognize it as sexual abuse or even grieve what happened to me until I was an adult. During that time, with God's empowerment, I began a healing process. It started with forgiveness, which was difficult and not something that came easy for me. Then one day, while I was praying, I asked God where He was during that difficult time. (Note: if abuse has occurred, it is recommended to begin visualizing the scene after the abuse has occurred so that you don't re-live the abuse again).

The picture I got was of the guy taking a knife and stabbing my heart. It was as if my heart was made of glass and shattered into a million pieces the day the sexual abuse occurred. I saw Jesus standing there crying and then lovingly picking up every last piece of my heart. He showed me the pieces and said, "You are not ready for them now, but I will keep them safe for you." I then saw him put all the pieces of my heart into a safe and lock it with a key.

He said to me, "Shelley, you have looked to your husband and to many other things to heal your heart, but I am the one who holds the key." Then, he looked at me and said, "Now, you are ready."

I then saw Jesus take out my broken heart and hold all the pieces in His hands. It was miraculously restored; all the broken pieces came back together to form a complete heart. He placed my restored heart back in my chest, but it was still not fully functioning and alive. I then watched him give me "CPR compressions" to get the blood flowing back through my heart again. The blood represents the Holy Spirit which now flows in and through my restored heart.

I can't fully explain it with words, but from somewhere deep inside I finally felt "whole" again. The next week in church we sang the song, "Love the Lord your God with all your heart, with all your strength, with all your mind…" and I sensed God saying to me, "Shelley, now you can love me with ALL your heart!" It wasn't an instant fix, but there was something that happened in my heart that day that started a deeper healing process for me.

Application

1. Pray and ask God for wisdom

If you are feeling broken hearted right now, pray and ask God for wisdom. You may want to consider seeing a Christian counselor (see the next chapter) or talking with your pastor. I have also included a list of books that have helped me in my journey of emotional healing in the appendix as a resource for you.

Chapter 18
Christian Counseling

Another tool God used to help me break free from pornography was Christian counseling. I do not remember exactly how long I went, but I do know that it was helpful to me in the process of healing from some wounds of the past.

I am not saying that Christian counseling is the answer to your problems. It is only a tool that God can use, just like all the other tools that I have shared with you. For some of you, counseling will not be an option, either due to finances or lack of availability of Christian counselors in your area. The great thing is that as followers of Christ, we already have a counselor available to us 24 hours a day, 7 days a week. His name is the Holy Spirit.

"And I will ask the Father, and he will give you another Counselor to be with you forever - the Spirit of truth. The world cannot accept him, because it neither sees him nor knows him. But you know him, for he lives with you and will be in you." John 14:16-17 (NIV 1984)

Some versions use the word "advocate," "helper," or "comforter" instead of the word *counselor*. It is the word *paraklētos* in the original Greek language which means "summoned, called to one's side, esp. called to one's aid. [1]

Isn't it good to know that the Holy Spirit's role is to come to your side to walk with you through your darkest days and to come to your aid? Many times, the Holy Spirit has been my only counselor as God has brought healing in certain areas of my life.

Yet, there have been other times that God has used a Christian counselor powerfully in my life. In my situation, they were reflective listeners and helped me process through all the emotions rolling around inside of me. When I was struggling with pornography, the counselor I saw helped me realize that I had some wounds from my past in regards to my relationship with my dad. My counselor led me through forgiving my dad and I wrote out a letter to him. I sensed God leading me to share this letter and the healing that God was doing in my life with him. This led to a healing and reconciliation in our relationship. At the time, my dad was a pastor. After this healing took place, he asked me to start meeting with him to pray with him every week. It was a beautiful time of bonding with my dad. It was just one of the positive things that came from my time of counseling.

Processing Our Emotions

As I was talking to my mom who has a degree in counseling, she suggested that we tend to go through the following four steps as we process our emotions. Unfortunately, most of us never get to step number four.

1. Circumstance / Trigger
2. Emotional response
3. Coping Mechanism

4. Re-anchor in God

Sometimes an emotional response to a circumstance or trigger can cause us to seek out coping mechanisms, like pornography and masturbation. What I have learned through my struggles is that we need to come to God and ask Him to help us work through our emotions as they come, to feel our emotions and then let them pass. Otherwise, they tend to pile up and build within us and can lead to coping behaviors.

It is also important to ask God to show us the triggers in our lives and how to recognize them. Then, ask Him to empower us to re-anchor in Him instead of just going with the wave of our emotions. In doing that, I believe we can go from #3, the emotional response, directly to #5, re-anchoring in God, bypassing all our coping mechanisms.

However, we cannot do it in our own strength. It is only possible when empowered by Christ.

"I am the vine; you are the branches. If a man remains in me and I in him, he will bear much fruit; apart from me you can do nothing." John 15:5

Application

1. Decide if counseling is for you

First of all, you need to decide if Christian counseling is what you need right now and a viable option for you financially and location-wise. Pray and ask God for wisdom in this step. Christian counseling is not for everyone, but it has definitely helped me. It has helped me to deal with issues from my past in a healthy and healing way.

Do not feel ashamed for reaching out to a counselor for help. Some people see it as a weakness or a bad thing to go to counseling. I see it as a temporary tool that God can use to help you heal.

I have a medical background with a degree in physical therapy, so God has given me this following illustration. I see Christian counseling in a similar way as a person who needs to use crutches after major surgery on their leg. The crutches simply help that person to walk until their leg heals enough that they can walk on their own again. In a similar way, Christian counseling is simply a tool to help us through a difficult time until we have experienced more healing and are able to "walk" on our own again.

2. Choose your Christian counselor

If you feel led to get some Christian counseling, there are many options available. First, I recommend checking with your insurance company to see what they will cover. At one point I was working for a hospital, and they offered 5 free visits to a counselor through their Employee Assistance Program (EAP). I did some research and found out one of the counselors was a Christian. Even though I had to drive 45 minutes for my appointment, the sessions were free and I knew they would be Christ-centered, so I encourage you to find out what your options are with your insurance.

Also, ask people you know for a referral. You can look in the phone book or research online, but a personal referral is often the best. Below you will find a list of places online to search for Christian counselors. I am not personally recommending any counselors from these places, simply passing on the resources to you.

- American Association of Christian Counselors (AACC)

The AACC has a listing of Christian counselors in the United States. You can search by certification and by state. http://www.aacc.net

- Focus on the Family

You can search their website to find counselors in the United States: http://referrals-loc.custhelp.com

- Christian Counseling Resource Directory

This is an online directory where you can research Christian counselors in your area.

www.christiancounselingresource.com

Sometimes you can also find a really good spiritual director to help you. A spiritual director does not have the same training as a counselor but can be a great reflective listener to help you process. I have benefited from seeing a spiritual director at a retreat center in the past.

3. Call, set up your first appointment and then go.

I know this seems obvious, but there was a time that I had identified a counselor to call, but it took me months to actually call and set up the appointment. Another time I almost backed out of going at all. I look back and can see now that there was a spiritual battle trying to keep me from getting the help and healing that I needed, so just do it!

Chapter 19
Journaling

I have to admit that I never grew up with a love for journaling. After I committed my life to Christ, many people recommended journaling as a way to connect with God and to keep a record of my spiritual growth. I tried. Honestly, I did, but no matter what I tried, I was not able to keep a consistent diary or journal. That is until I hit this crisis in my life and was desperate to be free of the stronghold of pornography.

I Was Surprised: Journaling Really Helped Me

Because I had not been a huge fan of journaling previously, I did not think it would help me, but it did. It helped me process some of the thoughts that were swirling around in my head. It was as if the same thoughts kept coming into my mind over and over without any resolution. I also felt like there was a bunch of radio stations being played at the same time in my mind and I could not make sense of any of them, but when I would journal, I could finally move past those initial jumbled thoughts and get deeper into what was really going on in my mind and emotions.

I also used journaling to write out my prayers to God, as well as keep a record of what I was learning. Believe it or not, my journals are now some of my most prized possessions. When I look back into my journals from the past, it helps me to remember all that God taught me during some of my darkest days. It also reminds me of all that God has done for me to bring me to where I am today.

In fact, my husband and I currently live in Colorado Springs and had to recently evacuate our home during the Waldo Canyon forest fire. I honestly did not know if we would be able to come back because the fire was so close to our home. We had to pack quickly when we evacuated and guess what I grabbed from all of our earthly belongings? I took a few picture albums as well as my box of mementos, including my journals. My journals are so valuable to me and something that cannot be replaced if lost in a fire. We ended up being able to return to our home without anything lost or damaged, but it reminded me once again about the value I place in my journals.

One particular book that I found helpful in the past, in regards to journaling, is called, *"My Healing Journey: An Interactive Guide to Spiritual Wholeness"* by Thom Gardner. In the book, the author provides space to journal your thoughts about what God is teaching you. You can find out more about this book and purchase a copy here:
www.bodyandsoulpublishing.com/healingjourney

Application:

1. Get a journal.

Some of my journals I have bought at Wal-Mart during their back to school sales for $0.25. You do not need anything fancy, just a blank notebook or journal to write down your thoughts.

2. Start writing out what God is teaching you.

One of the easiest things to do is to write out what God is teaching you. You could write down quotes, scriptures and illustrations you are learning. You can also write out your prayers to God.

3. Write to process your thoughts.

Are you frustrated, lonely or depressed but don't know why? Start journaling out your thoughts and ask God to reveal to you the core issue. You might be surprised to see that by journaling you are able to process your emotions much easier than just trying to think about it.

Note: I have had some women and teen girls tell me they are afraid someone will find their journal, therefore, they do not want to try it. In that case, I still recommend writing out your thoughts, but afterwards tearing the paper out of your journal and destroying it.   That way you can still process your emotions, without running the risk of someone else finding and reading it.

Chapter 20
Renewing Your Mind

As we begin to talk about renewing our minds, let me start by sharing an illustration. It has to do with weeds.

Let me ask you a question. What is important when weeding a garden? You need to be able to recognize which plants are weeds, right? Otherwise, you may uproot the good with the bad or allow certain weeds to continue to take root, thinking they are life giving, fruit bearing plants! Is not the same true in our lives in regards to our thoughts? We need to develop "weed recognition", the ability to recognize when the enemy is planting those weeds of lies into our lives. Even Jesus said that they will know you by your fruit (Matthew 7:15-20).

In my life, this has made a huge difference as I have learned how to renew my mind with God's truth instead of the lies of the enemy. In his book, "Waking the Dead," John Eldredge says,

> "Most of us simply try to 'put things behind us,' get past it, forget the pain as quickly as we can. Really – denial is a favorite method for coping for many Christians. But not with Jesus. He wants truth in the inmost being, and to get it there he's got to take us into our inmost being....to go with him into the deep waters of the heart, uncover the lies buried down there, and bring in the truth that

will set us free. Do not just bury it quickly; ask God what he is wanting to speak to."[1]

Often times those thoughts that keep coming up in your mind again and again, that tear you down instead of build you up, are lies from the enemy. In other words….."Stinkin' Thinkin,'" as my mom calls it.

Realize that those defeating thoughts are not from God, but from your enemy, Satan, who wants to destroy you and keep you captive. (John 8:43-45, John 10:10, Isaiah 61:1-4)

Some Examples of "Stinkin' Thinkin'":

- I am worthless.
- People I trust will hurt and betray me, therefore I cannot trust anyone.
- I am not as good as my friends.
- Something is wrong with me.
- I am ugly.
- I have to be perfect for people to like me.
- I am a failure and always mess up.
- Unless I have a man in my life, I am not complete.
- No one wants to be with me.

In place of those lies, begin to plant the seed of God's truth into your mind (2 Corinthians 10:5). Romans 12:2 says, "Do not be conformed to this world, but be transformed by the renewing of your mind, that you may prove what is that good and acceptable and perfect will of God."

It says we are transformed by the renewing of our minds and the only way to renew our minds is to change what goes into it.

A counselor once told me that our emotions are often indicators that there is something deeper going on within us. Therefore, when I get angry, upset, fearful, depressed, etc., I need to look deeper to see if the emotion is attached to a lie I believe. I was skeptical at first, but decided to give it a try. There would be days that I would feel as if a "dark cloud" descended over me emotionally. My emotions would then prompt me to reflect and see if I was believing a lie. Sometimes this "stinkin' thinkin'" was triggered by a circumstance of the day, and other times it was simply a thought that popped into my mind. However, over time God equipped me to recognize the lies from the enemy that I believed even quicker. Once I recognized the lie, I could then replace it with God's truth.

Did you know that one way people are trained to recognize counterfeit money is by studying the real thing? Therefore, one way we can get better at recognizing the lies is to know God's Truth in the Bible so well that we can quickly recognize those thoughts that are not from Him. Unfortunately, there is no shortcut for this step. The seed of truth may take time to grow. It is hard work, but definitely worth it!

One great way to renew your mind is to memorize Bible scriptures. I know it sounds boring, but think of it as a way to prepare for battle. I have found it to be one of the most effective ways for me to have victory over Satan in my life. Something else that has really helped me is praying God's word. If you are having difficulty overcoming a specific struggle in your life, I would recommend trying it. All you need to do is find scriptures that relate to that particular struggle and reword them into a prayer. Praying God's Word has changed my life during some really difficult times.

Starve the Flesh Feed the Spirit

> One evening an old Cherokee told his grandson about a battle that goes on inside people. He said, "My son, the battle is between two 'wolves' inside us all. One is evil. It is anger, envy, jealousy, sorrow, regret, greed, arrogance, self-pity, guilt, resentment, inferiority, lies, false pride, superiority, and ego. The other is good. It is joy, peace, love, hope, serenity, humility, kindness, benevolence, empathy, generosity, truth, compassion and faith."
>
> The grandson thought about it for a minute and then asked his grandfather: "Which wolf wins?"
>
> The old Cherokee simply replied, "The one you feed."
>
> *- Author Unknown*

The more we feed the flesh, the bigger this "monster" grows and the more damage is seen. It seems innocent at first. If you feel overwhelmed, do not! That is just another lie Satan is telling you to keep you from learning how to renew your mind with God's truth and find lasting freedom in Christ. I have felt the same way and have had great friends to help me.

Application

Take these practical steps to renewing your mind with God's truth: [2]

1. **Identify possible lies** in your life. Pray for God's wisdom and ask someone you trust to help you. Write them out on paper or a journal.

2. **Choose** one of the lies.

3. **Confess** the sin of believing this lie rather than the truth and living your life according to this lie.

4. When applicable, **forgive** your parents or family members that have passed down this lie to you. Also, forgive any others that have influenced you to form this lie.

5. **Repent**, asking for God's forgiveness for living your life based upon this lie.

6. **Reject the lie** and break its power from your life based on what Jesus did for you by dying on the cross.

7. **Plant God's truth** into your mind in place of the lie. Write out this truth.

8. **Receive this new truth** into your belief system as the replacement for the previously removed lie. (Repeat the above steps until you have gone through the entire list of lies).

9. **Pray:**

- that God would bring an end to the effects of this lie in your life.
- for this truth to be planted in your heart.
- that the Word of God already in your heart will be brought to the surface of your mind to use as a weapon against future defeating thoughts. (Ephesians 6)
- for the discipline to meditate on this new truth for at least 30 days.
- that the Holy Spirit would make you sensitive to falling back into old thought patterns and to be able to take captive any such thoughts.
- for new habits to be formed in your mind.

10. **Accountability** – As we talked about earlier, have someone you trust hold you accountable.

Examples of Replacing a Lie with the Truth

In the past I have taken the time to not only write out the lie that I believed, but also write out the truth of what God said about that situation. I then would write the truth on a notecard and carry it with me. Sometimes I have had to take out the card and re-read it multiple times throughout the day to fight the battle within my mind.

Here are just a few of mine that you can use as examples:

Lie: I cannot walk in consistent victory over sin.

Truth: I am not a slave to sin. Through Christ I have been set free from sin. (John 8:31-32, 36; John 14:6; Romans 6:6-7; Galatians 5:1; Hebrews 10:10)

Lie: I should not have to live with unfulfilled longings.

Truth: I will always have unfulfilled longings this side of heaven. The deepest longings of my heart cannot be filled by any created thing. If I will accept them, unfulfilled longings will increase my longing for God and for heaven. (Romans 8:23-25; Ephesians 3:11; Hebrews 11:13-16; Psalm 16:11, 73:25; Deuteronomy 8:3; Psalm 34:8-10, Philippians 3:20, 4:1)

Lie: God is not really enough.

Truth: God is enough. If I have Him, I have all I need. (Psalm 23:1, 73:23-26; Colossians 2:9-10)

Lie: When I am alone, I am lonely and rejected by others.

Truth: I can enjoy spending time by myself because my Father is always with me - He will never leave me. I am chosen, treasured and loved by Him. (Matthew 28:20; Deuteronomy 26:18)

Lie: I cannot trust God because He has let me down in the past.

Truth: God is faithful and has my best interests in mind, even when I can't understand His ways. He will help me begin to trust Him again. He wants me to trust Him and I want to trust Him. (Lamentations 3:5-6; Isaiah 55:9; Proverbs 3:5-6; Psalm 91:1-3)

Lie: I am not worthy of love.

Truth: The Father loves me completely, thoroughly and perfectly. There's nothing I can do to add or detract from that love. (Isaiah 54:10)

Lie: I am afraid of what the future holds.

Truth: God has plans for me - to prosper me and not to harm me, to give me a hope and a future. I can trust Him with my future. He is walking before me, preparing the way. (Jeremiah 29:11; Isaiah 43: 18-19)

Lie: I am ashamed of and regret my decisions and mistakes of the past. I can't forgive myself for what I have done.

Truth: I am free from condemnation. I am precious and honored in the eyes of my Father. I value God's opinion of me more than my past or what others think of me. My value comes from being the daughter of a King. (Romans 8:1-2; Isaiah 43:4; Romans 8:15-17)

I encourage you to come up with your own. Search the scriptures using tools like www.BibleGateway.com or www.YouVersion.com and find scriptures that relate to what you're going through. Re-word them into truths that you can post in your room, bathroom or car to carry with you, and repeat them until they replace the lies you have been believing!

Remember, this is just one step in your journey to finding freedom from pornography, but I can tell you from personal experience that it is powerful when you apply it to your life.

Chapter 21
Purity in All Areas

Many times freedom comes in stages. At times in my journey to become free from pornography, I felt like I was taking three steps forward and then two steps back. However, gradually, Christ began to do a new work in my heart that brought forward progress in my struggle against pornography.

Although Christ was healing my heart and helping me renew my mind, I still felt sexual temptations at times. Instead of desiring pornography, I began to have a stronger desire for the attention of men. Satan is often tricky in how he tries to keep us in bondage. Although I was not acting out in my struggle with pornography, I was flirting with men and having lustful thoughts in my mind. I would even go as far as saying that I had an emotional affair with another man during this time. Thankfully, it never went any further, but at this point in my life I was a married woman. Not good!

As I began to pray about this struggle, I realized that God wanted me to have purity in all areas of my life. This included the way I dressed and interacted with other men. In college my friends told me I was the "best flirt" and really knew how to get a guy's attention. Looking back, I am not proud of that fact and regret many of my actions. For many years, I used my power as a woman in a manipulative way with guys, to get my emotional needs met and to feel good about myself. This habit continued even after I was a married woman.

As I got dangerously close to having an affair, I realized that I needed to get serious about seeking purity in all areas of my life. God began to convict me of the way I dressed. Now, I was not dressing in an overly immodest way, showing cleavage or wearing miniskirts, but I definitely knew how to wear clothes that would show off my body and get a guy's attention.

So, I took on the task of going through my closet and evaluating my clothes one piece at a time. I would then decide what should stay and what should go. There are no hard and fast modesty "rules" in the Bible, but I knew instinctively the things that needed to go right away. Anything I was unsure of, I asked my husband for his opinion. If you are not married, you can also ask your dad or brother. My husband would either give me a thumbs up (it could stay) or a thumbs down (needed to go). I regret to say that I had a huge pile of clothes that had to go. Please note, I was not doing this to be legalistic and/or religious. I was making these changes in my life in order to walk a path of sexual purity in all areas of my life.

God also began to convict me of the way I flirted and interacted with guys. I would not have called it "flirting," but that is what it was. I am a very emotional person and can get emotionally attached to people very easily, so I realized that I needed to limit my personal conversations with men and also avoid time alone with men, especially if I felt a physical attraction to them.

God has changed me from the inside out. I still sometimes want to wear something that shows off my body, but I realize that ultimately, that is not the kind of attention I truly want. At times, I still want to capture a guy's attention and connect emotionally with him, but I recognize what is happening very quickly and bring it to God.

I have asked God for forgiveness for the many ways I have sinned against Him, and I have forgiven myself. I truly have repented and changed. It does not mean that I never struggle anymore or that I have "arrived," but I have received much healing and freedom through Christ.

I encourage you to never give up or lose hope if you feel like you are taking a few steps back. This happens to everyone. Realize that the enemy wants to derail you and keep you from having true freedom, but remember, God's power is much greater than Satan's and He wants to set you free.

I pray you find the same freedom that He has given me.

"It is for freedom that Christ has set us free. Stand firm, then, and do not let yourselves be burdened again by a yoke of slavery."

Galatians 5:1

Chapter 22
Connecting with God

We are all on a journey and each of us are in different places in our relationship with God. Some are just exploring who God is and how He can fit into their lives. Some have just begun a relationship with God, while others have been walking with God for a long time. Wherever you are on your journey, God is close by. He longs to have a relationship with you, but will not force you to spend time with Him.

However, I have found that meeting my needs through God is truly the way to stay free from my struggle with pornography. Just like many addictions, pornography and masturbation is just one way to fill a void in our hearts. What I found is that God wanted to fill that place with His presence in my life.

Feeling Far from God

I have to admit that I went through a time a few years ago where I felt far from God. It felt like there was a wall between God and me. I did not feel like praying and did not feel like reading my Bible. Maybe some of you can relate to feeling that way. Maybe you are in that place right now. For me, I had allowed some bitterness to take root in my heart as well as some unforgiveness towards some people who hurt me. They were people I trusted, which made it even harder.

Finally, I allowed God to come into my bitter and broken heart. The first step for me was forgiveness: forgiving those that hurt me, asking God's forgiveness, and finally forgiving myself. Then it felt as if that wall between God and me was finally removed! I truly had a desire to change. This is when I felt like I wanted to talk to God again through prayer and reading His Word. I actually felt like a sponge -- just soaking up my time with God.

Connecting with God Has Helped Me Stay Free from Pornography

In order to not be influenced by this culture and the media, I realized that I needed to spend more time with God than with the culture (including the media). There are several verses that talk about our need to stay connected to God and be a vessel for Him. Here are a few:

I am the vine; you are the branches. If a man remains in me and I in him, he will bear much fruit; apart from me you can do nothing.

John 15:5

I have been crucified with Christ and I no longer live, but Christ lives in me. The life I live in the body, I live by faith in the Son of God, who loved me and gave himself for me.

Galatians 2:20

But we have this treasure in jars of clay to show that this all-surpassing power is from God and not from us.

2 Corinthians 4:7

God gave me a picture of what it means to stay connected to Him. It is a picture of a hose connected to a faucet with water flowing through it, and a person watering dry plants.

In this illustration, I am the water hose, a vessel, and the only thing I need to do is stay connected to God, the faucet. When I am connected to my source (God), His water will flow through me. The water represents His Holy Spirit flowing through me, and Jesus is standing at the end of my hose guiding and directing the flow of the life-giving water to the dry places that need it the most. Just like Jesus guides and directs my life to impact those who are dry spiritually and need Him the most.

Are You Connected?

"As the hart pants and longs for the water brooks, so I pant and long for You, O God. *My inner self thirsts for God*, for the living God. When shall I come and behold the face of God?" Psalm 42:1-2 (AMP)

When Do You Feel Closest to God?

Whatever it is that helps you feel closest to God, do more of that activity. For me, it is prayer walks. For one of my friends, it is dancing in her room to worship music. For someone else, it might be listening to music, reading the Bible or a good book, spending time in nature, being silent, etc.

We are all different, so connect with God the way that works best for you. I pray that God fills your heart with His love and presence in a way that nothing else ever could.

Application

I have created a document, *"Four Ways to Connect with God"* which I encourage you to download to help you grow in your relationship with God (the link will open as a PDF):

www.bodyandsoulpublishing.com/connect

In Closing...

This is my prayer for you....

For this reason I bow my knees to the Father of our Lord Jesus Christ, from whom the whole family in heaven and earth is named, that He would grant you, according to the riches of His glory, to be strengthened with might through His Spirit in the inner man, that Christ may dwell in your hearts through faith; that you, being rooted and grounded in love, may be able to comprehend with all the saints what is the width and length and depth and height - to know the love of Christ which passes knowledge; that you may be filled with all the fullness of God.

Now to Him who is able to do exceedingly abundantly above all that we ask or think, according to the power that works in us, to Him be glory in the church by Christ Jesus to all generations, forever and ever. Amen.

Ephesians 3:14-21

APPENDIX
Appendix 1: Resources

There are resources to get help for pornography, but always remember that the most important part is to have the empowerment of the Holy Spirit. See the entire list of resources on our website:

www.bodyandsoulpublishing.com/pornresources

Books on Pornography

Free eBooks and Resources from Covenant Eyes
www.bodyandsoulpublishing.com/freepornbooks

Dirty Girls Come Clean by Crystal Renaud
www.bodyandsoulpublishing.com/dirtygirls

"Autobiography in Five Short Chapters" is a poem by Portia Nelson – This poem, also known as "Hole in My Sidewalk" has become widely known in many addiction recovery circles. I love the simple and yet powerful way that Portia describes recovery. Take a moment to read her poem now here: www.bodyandsoulpublishing.com/poem

Christian Books on Emotional Healing

Healing the Wounded Heart by Thom Gardner
www.bodyandsoulpublishing.com/woundedheart

My Healing Journey: An Interactive Guide to Spiritual Wholeness by Thom Gardner
www.bodyandsoulpublishing.com/healingjourney

Biblical Healing and Deliverance by Chester & Betsy Kylstra
www.bodyandsoulpublishing.com/biblicalhealing

Waking the Dead by John Eldredge
www.bodyandsoulpublishing.com/wakingthedead

Online Resources

Setting Captives Free: Setting captives free has a free 60 day Bible study for adults who struggle with pornography called, "Way of Purity: Freedom from the Bondage of Pornography (they have a course specifically for teens as well). You are assigned an accountability partner, so that is a great plus in getting help. I personally went through this course and recommend it. You can sign up for free here:
www.bodyandsoulpublishing.com/wayofpurity

X3pure.com: The ministry of XXXchurch.com has started a 30-day online program for women struggling with pornography. You can get more information about this program here:
www.bodyandsoulpublishing.com/x3pure

Covenant Eyes Free Webinars: Covenant Eyes offers many helpful webinars on pornography that you can watch for free here:

www.bodyandsoulpublishing.com/pornwebinars

Dirty Girls Ministry Community Signup: This is a private community forum that you can join for free to gain encouragement, accountability and hope in your journey to break free from pornography. We highly recommend that you sign up here:

www.bodyandsoulpublishing.com/dirtygirlscommunity

Captivated Documentary: Powerful documentary of the effects of media on our culture today.

www.bodyandsoulpublishing.com/captivated

Appendix 2: Compiled Statistics

Polled 241 American female Christians

Due to the small sample size, results from the survey are broken down by age brackets.

13 years old and under: 7%
14-18 years old: 49%
18-35 years old: 25%
35-50 years old: 15%
50 years old and over: 4%

Have you ever been involved in sexual conversations through texting (sexting) or the internet?

Overall:
41% - Yes
59% - No

The breakdown for each category:

13 and under:
39% - Yes
61% - No

14 – 18:
45% - Yes
55% - No

<u>18 – 35</u>:
54% - Yes
46% - No

Have you ever sent a naked picture of yourself to someone?

<u>Overall</u>:
18% - Yes
82% - No

The breakdown for each category:

<u>13 and under</u>:
11% - Yes
89% - No

<u>14 – 18</u>:
21% - Yes
79% - No

<u>18 – 35</u>:
25% - Yes
75% - No

Do you read romance novels that contain sexually explicit scenes?

<u>Overall</u>:
41% - Yes
59% - No

The breakdown for each category:

13 and under: 39%
14 – 18: 53%
18 – 35: 39%
35 – 50: 14%
50 and over: 10%

Have you ever been exposed to pornography before?

Yes – 73%
No – 27%

The breakdown for each category:
13 and under: 78%
14 – 18: 66%
18 – 35: 79%
35 – 50: 86%
50 and over: 80%

Note: the following questions apply only to the 73% of women that admitted to being exposed to pornography previously not the entire sample size.

How old were you when you were first introduced to pornography?

5-8 years old: 10%
9-11 years old: 15%
12-14 years old: 46%
15-17 years old: 15%

18-19 years old: 6%
Over 20 years old: 8%

So 71% of women who have been exposed to pornography were exposed to it before the age of 15.

How were you first introduced to pornography?

Internet search – 20%
Family – 14%
Friend – 14%
Magazine – 12%
TV/movie – 10%
Ads – 10%
Boyfriend – 9%
Internet (accidental) – 6%
Novels – 3%
Other – 3%

How often do you view pornographic material?

These are from the people that responded "yes" to having been exposed to pornography.

Daily: 5%
Weekly: 14%
Monthly: 9%
Every few months: 17%
Yearly or less: 10%
N/A: 45%

The last group most likely never looked at it again after first exposure.

How do you currently access pornography?

Internet received the largest response, followed by the phone.

Would you consider yourself addicted to pornography?
25%: Yes

Have you discussed this with anyone?
16%: Yes

Has your involvement with pornography led to other things (i.e. masturbation, sexual intercourse, etc.)?

59%: Yes

Have you ever felt hopeless in trying to overcome this addiction?

44%: Yes

About The Authors
Shelley Hitz

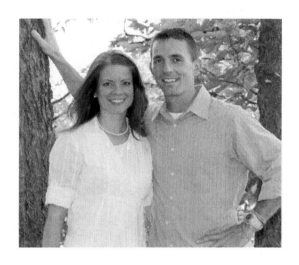

Shelley Hitz has been writing and publishing books since 2008, including the book she co-authored with S'ambrosia Curtis, "A Christian Woman's Guide to Breaking Free From Pornography: It's Not Just a Guy's Problem." You can download free resources and find out more at www.ChristianWomenandPorn.com.

Shelley has been ministering alongside her husband, CJ, since 1998. They currently travel and speak to teens and adults around the country. Shelley's main passion is to share God's truth and the freedom in Christ she has found with others. She does this through her books, websites and speaking engagements. Shelley's openness and vulnerability, as she shares her own story of hope and healing, will inspire and encourage you.

You can find out more about Shelley and connect with her online at www.ShelleyHitz.com or invite her to speak at your event at: www.ChristianSpeakers.tv.

S'ambrosia Curtis

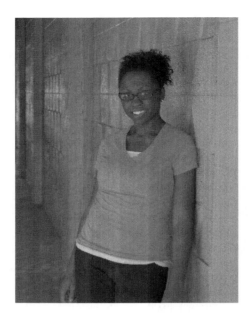

S'ambrosia Curtis is a graduate from Kansas State University, where she served on an InterVarsity leadership team for three years and developed a love for God and a heart for His people. Throughout college she was involved in various worship and prayer movements including two 24-hour campus-wide prayer vigils and an appearance in "Network" magazine with the founder of Burning Hearts, Becky Tirabassi. She currently teaches English and sociology to middle and high school students at Salina Christian Academy and leads worship at NorthPoint Church in Salina, KS. Her main objective for whatever she puts her hand to, is to bring glory to the name of Christ, that He may receive the reward of His suffering.

CJ and Shelley's Other Books:

21 Days of Gratitude Challenge
by Shelley Hitz

Unshackled and Free: True Stories of Forgiveness
by CJ and Shelley Hitz

The Forgiveness Formula: Finding Lasting Freedom in Christ
by CJ and Shelley Hitz

Fuel for the Soul: 21 Devotionals that Nourish
by CJ Hitz

Mirror Mirror…Am I Beautiful? Looking Deeper to Find Your True Beauty
by Shelley Hitz

Teen Devotionals…for Girls!
By Shelley Hitz and Heather Hart

Available on Amazon.com and Other Retailers

Love Getting Free Christian Books?

Get notified of our book promotions and download Shelley's eBook, "How to Find Free Christian Books Online" at:

www.bodyandsoulpublishing.com/freebooks

Special Thanks:

S'ambrosia would like to give a special thanks to Dana Dill for taking time out of her schedule to read and edit the manuscript. You've been incredibly influential in this process, Dana, and I'm looking forward to the next step God has for us!

References

Chapter 1: Pornography and Women

[1] Paul, Pamela. *Pornified: How Pornography is Transforming Our Lives, Our Relationships, and Our Families.* New York: Times Books, 2005. Print.

[2] Laaser, Mark R. (2010, March 29). Transforming the Brain [Review of the book *Wired for Intimacy: How Pornography Hijacks the Male Brain*]. *Christianity Today.* Web.

[3] Duke, Rachel B. "More women lured to pornography addiction." *The Washington Times* 11 July 2010. Web.

[4] Wetzstein, Cheryl. "Porn on the web exploding," *The Washington Times* 9 October 2003. Web.

[5] Ropelato, Jerry (n.d.) Internet Pornography Statistics. Web.

[6] Kastleman, Mark. "How Internet Pornographers Market to Women vs. Men. Web

[7] Ibid.

[8] McKay, Hollie. "Study: Sexual content in movies encourages earlier sex, more casual partners." *Fox News* 7 August 2012. Web.

[9] Pardun, Carol J., et. al. "Linking Exposure to Outcomes: Early Adolescents' Consumption of Sexual Content in Six Media." *Mass Communication & Society* 2005. Print.

[10] Ibid.

[11] Burger, David. (2011, September 12). "BYU study looks at the trend of increasing use of sexually explicit lyrics in music." Web.

[12] Hickey, Audrey. "Teen Magazines and Parents: Their Impact on Adolescent Female Sexual Scripts and Contraceptive Use." University of New Hampshire, n.d. Web.

Chapter 2: Pornography and Your Brain

[1] Pappas, Stephanie. (2012, April 19). "Watching porn may shut down part of your brain." *LiveScience.* Web.

[2] Ibid.

[3] Ibid.

[4] Kastleman, Mark B. (2007). *The Drug of the New Millennium: The Brain Science Behind Internet Pornography Use.* PowerThink Publishing.

[5] Ibid.

[6] Berne, E.C. (2008). *Online Pornography.* Detroit: Greenhaven. p. 61

[7] "Desensitization: A Numbed Pleasure Response." Online.

[8] Ibid.

[9] Ibid.

[10] "Pornography and Sex: Ted Bundy's Fatal Addiction." Online.

[11] http://digitalnaturopath.com/cond/C69153.html

[12] Ibid.

[13] "Masturbation Addiction: Find Lasting Freedom." Online.

[14] Kauflin, Bob. "Why Define Worship & Worship Defined." Online.

[15] Kinnear, Karen L. (2007). *Childhood Sexual Abuse*. ABC-CLIO Inc.

Chapter 3: Pornography and the Church

[1] http://www.purehope.net/stat.asp

[2] Means, Patrick. (1999). *Men's Secret Wars*. Revell.

[3] Berne, E.C. (2008). *Online Pornography*. Detriot: Greenhaven. p. 54

[4] N.A. (March 2005). *Christianity Today.*

[5] Ibid.

Chapter 12: Have You Opened the Door to the Enemy?

[1] The Barna Group. http://www.barna.org/barna-update/article/12-faithspirituality/260-most-american-christians-do-not-believe-that-satan-or-the-holy-spirit-exis

Chapter 17: When You Feel Broken Hearted

[1] Eldredge, John. Wild at Heart. Thomas Nelson, 2005. p.127-128.

Chapter 18: Christian Counseling

[1] Blue Letter Bible. "Dictionary and Word Search for paraklētos (Strong's 3875)". Blue Letter Bible. 1996-2012. 12 July

2012.www.blueletterbible.org/lang/lexicon/lexicon.cf
m?Strongs=G3875&t=KJV

Made in the USA
Lexington, KY
06 September 2013